Keto Diet for Beginners:

Keto Diet Guide for Beginners Code to Use Keto Aliments, Alkaline Plant and Vegetable to Fight Obesity and Weight Loss.

Table of Contents

Furthermore, the information that can be found within the pages described forthwith shall be considered both accurate and truthful when it comes to the recounting of facts. As such, any use, correct or incorrect, of the provided information will render the Publisher free of responsibility as to the actions taken outside of their direct purview. Regardless, there are zero scenarios where the original author or the Publisher can be deemed liable in any fashion for any damages or hardships that may result from any of the information discussed herein.

Additionally, the information in the following pages is intended only for informational purposes and should thus be thought of as universal. As befitting its nature, it is presented without assurance regarding its prolonged validity or interim quality. Trademarks that are mentioned are done without written consent and can in no way be considered an endorsement from the trademark holder.

Introduction

Congratulations on purchasing *Keto Diet for Beginners: An Ultimate Keto Diet Guide for Beginners Code to Use Keto Aliments, Alkaline Plant and Vegetable to Eliminate Obesity and Weight Loss Fast Improve Your Health Eating Healthy Food* and thank you for doing so.

The following chapters will discuss everything a beginner would need to know concerning the Keto Diet, and the impact such a diet would have on an individual's desire to lose weight and live a healthy life.

The first chapter is an introduction to the Keto diet. This chapter begins with a definition and an explanation of the keto diet. The chapter goes into detail to explain the science behind the diet, the advantages an individual committing to the diet will enjoy, and the overall health benefits of the diet.

Furthermore, the chapter explores the mechanism behind the diet, the common mistakes people make when trying to follow the diet, and the different types of keto diets out there. The chapter ends with an overview of the skills an individual would need to cultivate to gain success in this diet.

The second chapter is an in-depth explanation of the ketosis process. The chapter begins with tips on how an individual can start and get to a ketosis process. The chapter continues to explain the reasons keto is convenient, the process of testing for the ketosis process and the different ways people can use to eliminate the wrong type of fat.

The chapter concludes with the process that an individual can control his or her calories with low carb, an explanation of keto health, and the secret behind weight loss using keto.

The third chapter is a guide for someone who would want to start living the keto lifestyle. The chapter begins with encouraging an individual to consider the diet he or she is on, and then continues to point out the eating habits that such an individual would need to give up. The chapter continues to explain the food combinations people follow that are wrong in so many ways, and then concludes with a description of a healthy keto food combination.

The fourth chapter is about the keto shopping list. The chapter begins with an explanation of the different keto supplements an individual should look for in the market and the hormones balance in keto. The chapter continues to explain how keto in its totality can help with the fight against cancer, the benefits it has on the body, the brain, and the heart.

The fifth chapter is a breakdown of the different types of keto diet plans. The chapter begins with a description of the type of diet a beginner should subscribe to as he or she starts to get used to keto. The chapter continues to explain the basic plan, it explains the snacks an individual can take, and even the plan one would need to follow if he or she were fasting. The chapter concludes with the keto plans for vegetarians and vegans.

The sixth chapter is the place to get to for anyone who is interested to find out as much as he or she can concern keto cycling. The chapter begins with a definition of keto cycling, it explains the specific aspects of the cycle program and explains the benefits of keto cycling. The chapter concludes with distinguishing between keto cycling and carb cycling and then takes you on a journey to discover whether keto cycling is good for you.

There are plenty of books on this subject on the market, thanks again for choosing this one! Every effort was made to ensure it is full of as much useful information as possible, please enjoy it!

Chapter 1: Introduction to Keto Diet

At the beginning of every year, and every day in between, people hear about a new diet, detox plan, or gym membership that promises to be the secret to a successful year or a healthy life. Sometimes, it seems like the whole world is trying to get rid of a few extra pounds as fast as possible. Often people are willing to try anything that sounds remotely promising.

Enter the keto diet. This diet plan is one of the hottest trends currently. Interestingly, its origins date back to the 1920s as a treatment plan for childhood epilepsy. Due to its overwhelming popularity and success rate, many people still use it to deal with this condition today.

According to some studies, people who follow this diet experience up to 40% fewer epileptic seizures. Its use, however, is more common in the generally healthy population seeking to get more out of life or drop a few pounds. This diet plan promises a wide range of benefits from increased mental focus to faster weight loss.

The keto diet aims to decrease insulin and blood sugar levels by shifting the body's metabolism to burn fat more effectively to generate energy, which leads to the production of ketones.

In addition, proponents of this diet plan insist that it can help people lose weight quite fast, which is one of the reasons why it is so popular.

However, to determine whether this diet plan is good for them, people need to learn as much as possible about the keto diet. They need to determine whether science backs it before joining the cause and adopting it into their lifestyle.

What Is the Keto Diet Plan?

The word keto comes from the fact that this diet plan drives the body to produce ketones, which are tiny energy/fuel molecules. The body turns to this fuel source when the level of blood sugar is low. The human brain is a constantly hungry organ that needs a lot of energy, which is understandable given the work it does every second. However, it cannot run on fat; rather, it needs glucose or ketones.

This diet plan consists of consuming food that is low in carbohydrates, moderate in protein, and significantly high in fat. Actually, according to some keto diet variations, the fat content should make up to 80% of a person's daily calories. The carbohydrates, on the other hand, should be less than 5% of the calories. Protein should contribute between 15% and 20% of the calories.

It is easy to see why many people are apprehensive about this diet plan. The keto diet drastically departs from the generally accepted macronutrient distribution of 10% to 35% fat, 45% to 65% carbs, and 20% to 35% protein. However, the most important aspect of this diet is the normal and natural process known as ketosis.

The healthy human body runs quite well on the glucose produced when the body burns or breaks down carbohydrates. Actually, the human body prefers to generate energy through the breakdown of carbohydrates. However, when a person is hungry or cutting back on carbohydrates, his/her body will seek other sources of energy.

Fat is an alternative source of energy for the body. When a person's blood sugar is low because he/she is not feeding his/her body with carbohydrates, his/her cells will release fat and flood the liver. Consequently, the liver will turn the fat into ketone bodies, which the body will use as its secondary energy source.

In other words, the ketogenic diet aims to substitute the body's primary sources of energy with fats. Actually, this process is surprisingly efficient, which is why it leads to weight loss and other health benefits. Another subtle benefit of this diet plan is that one will have a constant supply of energy and feel hungry less often.

Consequently, one will feel focused and sharp all day. As stated earlier, the keto diet helps decrease insulin and blood sugar levels. Sugar, however, is the brain's main fuel or food. Fortunately, ketones produced by the liver from fat will feed the brain. Most people who follow this diet plan insist it is quite safe.

Nevertheless, the ketogenic diet is still controversial. Actually, three groups of people should keep away from this diet. These are breastfeeding women, people with high blood pressure taking antihypertensive medication, and people with diabetes who take insulin. Before adopting this diet, people in these situations should seek their doctors' advice.

People on a keto diet force their bodies to run on fat, essentially, their bodies burn fat 24 hours a day, seven days a week, as long as they are following this diet plan religiously. The fastest way to get the body into a state of ketosis is through fasting. However, it is extremely difficult to fast for several days.

This is where the keto diet comes in handy. This diet plan helps the body reach this state surprisingly fast, and people can adopt and follow it indefinitely. A typical ketogenic diet consists of foods such as butter, meat, cheese, fish, eggs, heavy cream, avocado, oils, seeds, nuts, and low-carb green veggies.

Looking at this list, one will notice that it does not include people's favorite carbohydrate-rich foods such as fruits, grains, cereals, rice, milk, beans, sweets, potatoes, and even some veggies.

The Science of Keto

Every year, new diet fads rise and fall with little to commend them. Nothing new there; however, the keto diet has been around for a remarkably long time and continues to gain popularity because of the science behind it. Many prominent medical professionals believe in the benefits of ketosis, which is reason enough for one to take a closer look at this diet.

After years of trying any weight loss diets, most overweight individuals come to believe that nothing makes a difference. They only lose some weight if they consume fewer calories than they used to, but when they do this, then they feel hungry all the time, which causes them to binge eat on certain occasions. When such individuals learn about the ketogenic diet, few can resist its attraction.

The concept behind this diet plan makes a lot of sense. The weirdly named ketone bodies are tiny molecules that serve as the natural back-up fuel supply for the body when glucose is in short supply. As stated earlier, people normally enter ketosis when they starve themselves for several days at a time.

Ketosis is the state where ketone bodies build up in the bloodstream. When the body reaches ketosis, metabolism switches to fat-burning to convert accumulated fat molecules into ketone bodies, which help power the brain and muscles. Being in a state of ketosis, therefore, sounds like an awesome way to get rid of excess fat.

Not eating for days, on the other hand, is not something most people would be willing to do. Fortunately, the keto diet seems to be the answer to this dilemma. People do not need to starve themselves to reach ketosis. Instead, all they need to do is drastically reduce the carbohydrates in their diet, and this includes refined carbs, complex carbs, as well as starches.

When the body lacks a source of glucose, it has to go into a state of ketosis since the brain needs fuel in the form of either glucose or ketone bodies to function and survive. Therefore, no matter how much fat or protein one eats, the body will still need to break down fat to ketone bodies to produce the fuel it needs.

As earlier stated, there are many variations of the keto diet. All of them, however, aim to switch the body's metabolism to ketosis. Actually, the keto diets doing the rounds out there are not the only ones or the first to do that. The Atkins diet, for example, rose to prominence a few decades ago and helped many people lose weight.

The Atkins diet, in reality, is another variation of the keto diet since it removes carbohydrates from the diet and substitutes them with protein. Interestingly, followers of this diet discovered that they felt less hungry than they feared, which means that the calories from increased protein intake made the feel satisfied for longer.

When one is feeling full, one will eat less, which will translate to significant weight loss. The Atkins diet, however, has certain side effects for people who follow it for an extended period. The most troubling of these side effects is its impact on the balance of nitrogen from the consumption of too much protein.

For example, there is an increased risk of dehydration for those who adhere to the Atkins diet. In serious cases, the need to get rid of excess nitrogen as urine leads to the formation of kidney stones. In a certain sense, the keto diet is the 21st-century version of the Atkins diet. Instead of replacing carbohydrates with protein, the keto diet replaces them with fats.

The regimen of a typical Atkins diet consisted of less than 5% of calories from carbohydrates, 25% from fats, and about 75% from protein. The modern keto diet regimen, in contrast, suggests 25% of calories from protein, less than 5% from carbohydrates, and about 75% from fats.

Since the intake of protein in the keto diet is the same as the recommended protein intake in a typical balanced diet, it neatly sidesteps the side effects resulting from nitrogen imbalance. However, the recommended fat intake in the keto diet is a huge concern for many people.

It seems more than a bit ironic that it advocates for people who want to get rid of excess fat to include more fats in their diet. To many people, it seems quite unhealthy. To help understand this conundrum, consider the case if the lipid profiles of the brave individuals who explore and cross the Antarctic on foot while dragging sleds packed with food and supplies.

To achieve this feat, they need to take food with a very high calorie to weight ratio. Essentially, this means eating a lot of butter. It takes several months to cross the continent on foot, which means living on an all-butter diet for months. Interestingly, after months on this diet, the level of bad cholesterol in their bodies, known as LDL-cholesterol, actually decreases significantly.

This may surprise many people, but it is not as surprising as it sounds. When the body goes into ketosis, it moves fats towards the liver, where the transformation of fats into ketone bodies happens, which is the work of HDL-cholesterol. Usually, LDL-cholesterol transports excess fat from the liver to deposits in different parts of the body.

Essentially, this type of cholesterol moves fat in the opposite direction. In ketosis, therefore, no matter how much fat one is consuming, one will have a lipid profile usually considered healthier. In other words, one will have lower LDL and higher HDL, which is quite remarkable.

However, as discussed earlier, one of the benefits of following the Atkins diet was reduced feelings of hunger due to the sustaining power of protein. People often wonder how the keto diet can achieve this without increasing the protein content of their diet. As it turns out, reduced hunger stems from the state of ketosis itself.

In a certain sense, it might not matter how one achieves this state. Therefore, theoretically, science seems to back up the modern keto diet. However, it would be somewhat interesting to imagine how it would feel to follow the keto diet in place of the commonly touted, calorie-deficient, low-everything diet.

Consider a man weighing 195 pounds on a 5-foot, 9-inch frame at the beginning of the year. This would put his body mass index at about 30, which is quite close to being obese. Anyway, on the first day of the year, he reads about the keto diet, does some research, and decides to try it.

He purchases one of the deliciously sounding cookbooks from Amazon and begins the keto journey. His intake of carbohydrates immediately falls below 5%, which means, among other things, eating a rib-eye steak topped with chili-butter, followed with cheese and scrambled eggs in the morning. This sounds somewhat awesome.

Anyway, people who believe that fats are an important ingredient in great tasting food should find the keto diet quite appealing and easy to follow. This man usually works out for 30 minutes each day on a rowing machine. To improve the effectiveness of his new diet, he decides to increase his workout time to 45 minutes.

This workout will help get rid of excess carbohydrates in his body stored as glycogen in the liver, which will release quickly to power his muscles. Within 2 days, he reaches ketosis. Using urine dipsticks, he determines that his ketone body level indicates a state of deep ketosis.

The level of ketone bodies stayed constant for more than a month while he enjoyed the culinary delights of meals such as cream pork stroganoff accompanied by zucchini ribbons sour cream and avocado dressings, and burgers. Essentially, he was eating three fat-rich meals each day.

In this example, it is important to look at the benefits he enjoyed before looking at any disadvantages. Once he went into a state of ketosis a few days on, he founds that he was never hungry. Essentially, he stopped snacking between meals as he usually did. Actually, he found himself thinking less about eating.

Soon, missing lunch altogether by accident became something quite normal. There was a significant improvement in his focus and concentration as well, in addition to having more energy, which also increased his productivity. In other words, using his back-up batteries, which are the tiny ketone bodies, seemed to be better than using carbohydrates for fuel.

There is a good reason why this might happen, especially for a chubby individual like the person in this example. Essentially, the ketone levels never decline. By contrast, when people eat carbohydrate-rich foods, the metabolism system immediately turns the excess carbohydrates into fat. In a sense, it stores it for a rainy day.

Therefore, after eating a carbohydrate-rich meal, a person's blood glucose level starts to decrease a few hours after, which triggers feelings of hunger and the urge to eat again. In addition, it also triggers a sense of declining concentration and energy, which 'carbavores' and late afternoon dippers know so well.

Going back to the hypothetical man in the example above, eating less actually led to a significant loss of weight. For this example, based on a testimonial from the real individual, he lost 10 pounds in less than a month, mostly from unhealthy-looking and unattractive fat deposits on his body.

According to his testimonial, his waistline decreased by two notches, which is twice as much as his previous diet achieved by keeping hi constantly hungry. In addition, the keto diet brought other unexpected benefits as well. The amount of plaque on his teeth, for example, reduced quite significantly, maybe because carbohydrates need to feed off dietary carbohydrates.

When it comes to the downside of the keto diet, at least according to him, there were just a few. The first is about staying away from carbohydrates, keeping them below 5% proved to be quite challenging after a couple of weeks. He had to check the content of carbohydrates in everything he ate, which was difficult because he found them in almost everything he chose to eat.

Eating out was also a challenge, not to mention having to attend dinner parties at a family member or friend's house unless they were unusually accommodating. As a result, planning and preparing food took on a new level of significance and demand for his resources and time than previously.

Secondly is the issue of accurate portion control. Since the keto diet includes high-fat meals with high-calorie content, he often feared he would unintentionally consume too many calories. To lose weight people need to eat fewer calories than they need. Even the ketogenic diet cannot break this law.

The last downside was a bit easier to avoid. While following the keto diet, it is difficult to get enough fiber mainly because most of the fiber sources commonly available also contain carbohydrates. Essentially, since fiber is an indigestible or insoluble carbohydrate polymer, it naturally contains digestible carbohydrates. His solution was to take a fiber supplement.

If this man were to conduct an experiment to determine the impact of eating some carbs after following a carbohydrate-free diet for a month, just a small portion of carbohydrates would immediately kill ketosis. He would then need to re-establish ketosis after one moment of weakness. Following the keto diet, therefore, requires Zen-like discipline.

This experiment shows that ketosis is difficult and slow to establish, but very easy to turn off. Scientists call this phenomenon hysteresis. There are good reasons for this. Although carbohydrates and glucose good sources of fuel, they can damage the proteins that make up the body's tissues and cells.

When the levels of glucose go up too much, this tissue and cell damage may be irreversible, which can happen in diabetes. To prevent this from happening, the body produces insulin as soon as the levels of blood glucose start to go up. Insulin limits glucose levels in the blood by instructing the liver to turn excess glucose into fat.

In the process, however, insulin kills ketosis, which is why ketosis ends so quickly when people following the keto diet slip up. Nowadays, there is unlimited availability of calories.

The body stores every ounce of excess carbohydrates as fat. Without establishing ketosis, the body will not re-assess these fat deposits when glucose runs out; instead, one will simply feel hungry. With fast-food joints around every corner, it is extremely tempting to refuel with carbohydrates again.

As stated earlier, one reason why people lose weight while on a keto diet is that feelings of hunger go way down, which forces more fat out of fat deposits for energy than the fat that goes in. Without spikes in insulin, the body takes advantage of leptin-induced satiety ore easily.

The keto diet also helps people wean off dopamine addiction caused by spiking blood sugar, which raises HDL and reduces LDL and triglycerides in obese people. However, people who want to try the keto diet should first discuss it with their doctor to determine whether it is good for them.

Benefits of Keto Diet

The keto diet is one of the most popular diets today, which is why there are more than a million Google searches every month for this diet. Some of the reasons for its popularity include:

1. It Helps People Lose Weight

Initially, weight loss results from loss of water because of the drastic reduction in carbohydrate intake. The keto diet also encourages people to consume foods rich in fat and cut back on carbohydrates, sugar, and refined carbohydrates. This will lead to a constant supply of energy and fewer sugar highs and crashes.

Actually, the first thing people on this diet report is having steady energy and not needing to snack all the time due to waning energy. Essentially, the keto diet often lowers the desire to eat and leads to fewer hunger pangs. If one is not hungry all the time, one will eat less, which will lead to weight loss.

Interestingly, although the keto diet is high in fat content, it is often more effective when it comes to helping people lose weight than a low-fat diet. However, it is not right for everyone. While it may lead to short-term weight loss, it is extremely difficult to follow.

2. Treating Epilepsy in Kids

The only clear and proven health benefit of the keto diet is its ability to reduce epileptic seizures in kids. In fact, since 1920, doctors have been using it therapeutically for this very purpose. Experts recommend the keto diet for children suffering from certain conditions, such as Rett syndrome or Lennox-Gastaut syndrome, and do not respond to medication for seizure.

The Epilepsy Foundation suggests that the ketogenic diet can decrease the number of seizures kids have by up to 50%, with about 10% to 15% of children becoming seizure-free. The foundation also notes that this diet can also be beneficial for adults who suffer from epilepsy, although it is quite difficult and restrictive to stick with.

3. May Improve Heart Health

When a person follows the keto diet in a healthy manner, it can improve the health of his/her heart by reducing bad cholesterol. In addition, this diet also increases the levels of HDL-cholesterol, which is good cholesterol.

4. Reduces Acne

There are many different forms of acne, and some may have a connection to blood sugar and diet. A diet rich in refined and processed carbohydrates, for example, can alter the bacteria in the gut and dramatic fluctuations in the levels of blood sugar, which can have a negative effect on skin health. Limiting carbohydrates intake; therefore, can help reduce some forms of acne.

5. Metabolic Syndrome

Limited research suggests that adults suffering from the metabolic disease can benefit from the keto diet because it can help them get rid of more body fat and weight, compared to people who eat a diet heavy in added sugars and processed foods.

6. Type 2 Diabetes

In September 2016, the Journal of Obesity and Eating Disorders published research suggesting that the keto diet could be helpful to people with type 2 diabetes and lead to improvements in the levels of HbA1c. However, it is important to understand that it can also lead to low blood sugar levels, also called hypoglycemia, if the patient also takes medication to lower his/her blood sugar.

7. Bipolar Disorder

The keto diet may be a mood stabilizer for individuals with type 2 bipolar disorder. According to a study published in the journal Neurocase in October 2012, in certain cases, it may be more effective than medication.

8. Obesity

According to one study published in the journal Endocrine in December 2016, obese people on a low-calorie keto diet lose ore inflammatory belly fat as compared to those on a normal low-calorie diet. In addition, according to a February 2018 article published in the journal Nutrition and Metabolism, this diet may also help maintain a lean body mass during weight loss.

9. Alzheimer's Disease and Dementia

An article in the journal Neurobiology of Aging published in February 2013 suggested that higher-risk older adults on a ketogenic diet experienced significantly better memory functioning after one and a half months.

Certain experts in the field of Alzheimer's, such as the director of the Alzheimer's Prevention Clinic at Weill Cornell Medicine and New York Presbyterian, Richard Issacson, MD, suggest low-carbohydrate diets as one of the ways to delay brain aging, and maybe even Alzheimer's, which is a form of dementia.

10. Parkinson's Disease

Since people with this condition tend to have a higher risk of developing dementia, experts like Robert Krikorian, Ph.D., a professor of clinical psychiatry, are conducting studies looking at whether inducing dietary ketosis can preserve cognitive functioning. Only time and more research will tell.

11. Certain Forms of Cancer

Some studies, such as one published in the journal Oncology in November 2018; suggest that doctors should use the ketogenic diet in conjunction with radiation and chemotherapy to treat certain forms of cancer.

However, to determine whether this diet can play a helpful role in cancer therapy, scientists need to conduct more studies. More importantly, without a doctor's consent, patients should not use the keto diet as a stand-alone treatment for any disease.

12. Polycystic Ovary Syndrome

Women with this infertility condition have a higher risk of developing obesity and diabetes. This is why some medical professionals recommend the ketogenic diet. However, researchers need to conduct long-term research on the safety of using the keto diet to deal with this condition.

- **Other Unexpected Benefits**

Some researchers suggest the possibility of gaining several other unexpected benefits from the keto diet. These findings, however, are preliminary and require more research. These include:

1. The diminishment of anxiety and depression

2. A healthier liver

3. A fall in inflammation markers

4. Sound sleep

Advantages of The Keto Diet

In the beginning, the ketogenic diet can be quite overwhelming. Before people give it a go, they need to understand what it involves, how the diet works, and, most importantly, what doctors and nutritionists think about the ketogenic diet. According to many people who follow the keto diet plan, it provides impressive results within a very short time.

Research also suggests that the keto diet may even improve workout performance in athletes and help them lose body fat while maintaining muscle mass. However, it is important to note that conflicting evidence exists to support these claims. Some experts, for example, express concerns about the sustainability of this diet plan, as well as its long-term effects on the body.

Some of the common advantages of the keto diet include:

1. Quick weight loss

2. Tons of online recipes and resources

3. Ability to boost satiety

4. Improved athletic performance in certain people

5. Reduced abdominal fat

6. Ay improve health markers like cholesterol levels, triglyceride, and blood pressure

Mechanism of Keto Diet

The keto diet restricts the intake of proteins and especially carbohydrates while encouraging the consumption of fat. For several decades, doctors have been using this diet plan in the management and treatment of drug-resistant epilepsy. This is because its action mechanism leads to changes in ketone levels and other substances, thereby reducing the frequency of seizures.

- **Seizure Pathophysiology**

The brain has a complex network of neurons that transmit signals and nerve impulses. These transmitters play a critical role in the dissemination of these nerve impulses, which carry messages across the neuron synapse. Neurotransmitters are inhibitory or excitatory based on their effect on the triggering of impulses.

A common excitatory neurotransmitter is a glutamate, which aids the distribution of impulses. On the other hand, GABA serves to inhibit nerve impulses. Any imbalance between the brain's neurotransmitters causes a seizure, especially due to the firing of too many nervous messages and over-excitement of the nerves.

Therefore, GABA helps to control the frequency of epileptic seizures, while anticonvulsant medication helps to boost inhibitory neurotransmitters. Scientists do not know the keto diet's precise mechanism; however, they propose several possible explanations.

Many changes take place in the brain and body because of the keto diet. However, science is yet to identify the change that leads to the anticonvulsant effect. That said, the action mechanism of most pharmacological anticonvulsant medication is similarly mysterious.

The most important aspect of the keto diet is the drastic restriction of carbohydrates from the diet. To compensate for this reduction, the conversion of fatty acids into sources of fuel takes place through oxidation in the mitochondria. The lack of carbohydrates in the diet leads to the absence of glucose.

Acetone, acetoacetate, and hydroxybutyrate, which are ketone bodies, synthesize and pass through the blood-brain barrier to provide an alternative energy source for the brain. Scientists think they possess anticonvulsant properties needed to prevent seizures in test animals.

The propagation of nerve messages and stabilization of neurons may happen because of the ketone bodies' efficiency as a source of fuel. As the body adapts to the conversion of fat to produce ketone bodies for energy, the increase in the number of mitochondria takes place.

Both the keto diet and pharmacological anticonvulsants work because of their ability to suppress seizures. Unlike anticonvulsant medication, however, the keto diet seems to have anti-epileptogenic properties and the ability to hinder the progress of epilepsy, at least according to a study of rats.

There are several other theories about the keto diet's action mechanism, such as hypoglycemia, electrolyte changes, and systemic acidosis, which is increased blood acidity. However, science is yet to prove the accuracy of most of these theories. In addition, some evidence suggests that these hypotheses may not have anything to do with the diet's mechanism.

Within the past twenty years or so, interest in determining the therapeutic mechanism of the keto diet has been growing steadily. Fortunately, modern advances in the scientific and medical fields are yielding critical insight into the biochemical basis of many brain functions, both pathologic and normal.

Some of the metabolic changes likely connected to the keto diet's anticonvulsant properties include increased bioenergetics reserves, increased fatty acid levels, reduced glucose levels, and ketosis.

According to some experts in the field of neuroscience, some of the effects induced by the keto diet may include GABA neurotransmission and enhanced purinergic, sensitive potassium channel modulation, and boosted brain-derived neurotrophic factor expression because of glycolytic limitation.

More importantly, in addition to its use as an anticonvulsant, the keto diet may also promote neuroprotective properties, which can help boost the clinical potential of the diet as an illness-prevention approach or intervention.

Since scientific evidence proves that changes in diet can trigger a wide range of complex metabolic alterations, future scientific research should reveal a more detailed framework for the keto diet mechanism in action, which will allow for the formulation of an improved offering with fewer side effects for a wide range of physical disorders.

Some scientists proposed the modulation of the levels of biogenetic monoamine as a plausible action mechanism for the anticonvulsant properties of the keto diet. The specific workings underlying such properties, however, remain unclear. Norepinephrine levels in test animals seem to show an increase in rats consuming this diet.

When researchers inhibited the transport of norepinephrine, there was no observable benefit from the keto diet. This seems to suggest the need for a noradrenergic system for the neuroprotective properties of the ketogenic diet to take place.

From this brief discussion, it is clear to see the complexity of the keto diet's mechanism of action.

Common Mistakes of Keto

The hottest diet last year, which is the ketogenic diet, is only gaining momentum this year. It attracts more than one million searches on Google each month, which is a testament to its popularity. However, this popularity tends to make people who want to try it out make various mistakes.

Unfortunately, people tend to jump headlong into any weight loss and wellness diet that promises amazing results without doing adequate research to determine whether the diet is right for them. This is also true when it comes to the keto diet. It is difficult to know what to expect when one decides to follow the keto diet without proper research.

The most important thing to understand about this low-carb, high-fat diet is that it is extremely restrictive; therefore, getting it right can be quite difficult. For example, in addition to the obvious carbohydrates, people who want to adopt this diet need to avoid starchy vegetables and limit grains, fruits, sweets, and juices.

In addition, they will need to bulk up on fats, according to the recommended keto food list. By doing this, they will go into ketosis within a very short time, which, as discussed earlier, is the metabolic state that forces their bodies to burn fat to generate fuel, instead of burning carbohydrates. In most cases, this will speed up their weight-loss goals.

Since carbohydrates are in just about everything people eat today and fats come in several different forms, it is easy to make mistakes, especially if one does not know much about the ketogenic lifestyle. At this point, it is important to understand that not all fats are healthy.

To live the keto lifestyle safely, one needs to understand the common mistakes people make, including:

1. **Increasing Fat Intake and reducing Carbohydrate Intake too Quickly and too Much**

One day, one is eating cereal in the morning, sandwiches at lunch, and pasta for dinner. Suddenly, having decided to adopt the keto diet, one will need to consume less than 20 grams of carbohydrates every day, based on the starting amount recommended by the keto diet. This is harder to achieve than it sounds.

A medium apple, for example, contains approximately 25 grams of carbohydrates. This is a good point of reference for people who decide to follow the keto diet. Essentially, this diet requires drastic dietary and lifestyle changes. Therefore, it is important to ease into the diet. Before adopting this diet fully, people should begin by decreasing their carbohydrates intake gradually, instead of doing it cold turkey.

2. Failing to Drink Adequate Water

When most people start weight loss or wellness diets, including the keto diet, they tend to focus on what they are eating and forget about what they are drinking. People on the ketogenic diet have an increased risk of dehydration due to the extreme decrease in their carbohydrate intake.

This can easily lead to a shift in electrolyte and fluid balance. The body stores carbohydrates along with water; therefore, as the deposits of carbohydrates in the body run dry, excess water in the body also depletes. In addition, the body gets rid of excess ketones through urine, which depletes sodium and water from the body.

Therefore, it is important to drink a lot of water to prevent dehydration. When one wakes up, for example, one should drink a glass of water and sip water regularly throughout the day, which will help one reach the goal of drinking half of one's body weight in ounces of water every day.

3. Failing to Prepare for the Keto Flu

As one's body transitions from a carb engine to a fat engine, one might experience the keto flu, which comes with flu-like symptoms such as fatigue, body aches, nausea, and cramps. This often happens during the first couple of weeks; however, these symptoms do not affect everyone who adopts this diet.

People who lack knowledge about the keto diet and fail to prepare themselves for these symptoms often think there is something very wrong, which makes them give up on the diet altogether.

However, such people can overcome these symptoms by planning their prepping and meal preparation in advance. It is also wise to eat foods rich in sodium, magnesium, and potassium, in addition to drinking water to help deal with any negative symptoms of this diet.

Other common mistakes people make when they decide to adopt the keto diet include:

- Failing to eat foods rich in omega-3 fatty acids

- Failing to salt their food adequately

- Failing to consult their doctor about the diet and trying to do it alone

- Failing to pay attention to their vegetable intake

- Focusing on the carbohydrate intake and forgetting about the quality of food

- Drinking too much dairy

- Snacking too much

- Being obsessive about the scale

- Not sleeping enough

Types of Keto Diet

Since the end goal of different variations of the keto diet is the same, these variations share certain similarities, the most notable of which is high dietary fats and low carbohydrates. To put together the right diet, it is important to speak to a doctor or dietician who will give one personalized guidance and advice based on one's individual needs.

Some of the most common types of keto diets include:

1. The common keto diet composed of 20% protein, 70% to 75% fat, and 5% to 10% protein

2. The extremely low carbohydrate keto diet with less than 5% carbohydrate content

3. The well-formulated keto diet with macronutrients of carbohydrates, protein, and fat that meet the requirements or standards of the keto diet

4. The medium-chain triglycerides keto diet

5. Calorie-restricted keto diet

6. Cyclical keto diet

7. Targeted keto diet

8. The high protein keto diet

Skills for Success in Keto Diet

The keto diet can be extremely difficult to start and maintain since it radically departs from the way people eat these days. The typical American diet, for instance, is high in both processed foods and carbohydrates. The keto diet, however, involves putting the body into a state of ketosis to force it into burning fat for energy.

Some of the skills needed to follow and maintain the keto diet include:

1. Knowing the foods to avoid and eat

2. Understanding one's relationship with fat

3. Improving one's cooking skills

4. Drinking bulletproof coffee, which is one of the best ketogenic-friendly drinks

5. Seeking support from family members and friends

The ketogenic diet or keto, in short, went viral last year. Actually, 2018 was the year of the ketogenic diet. Even today, it shows no signs of slowing down. The internet has tons of guides about this diet because it is somewhat difficult to follow and maintain. There are many different variations of the keto diet plan on the internet. Therefore, it is important to talk to a doctor or dietician before embarking on the ketogenic journey.

Chapter 2: What Is the Ketosis Process?

If you have searched for ways to lose weight, you might have come across this word Ketosis. Ketosis refers to a natural metabolic process whereby the body burns stored fats to get energy when there is not enough supply of glucose or carbohydrates in the body. You can achieve this by observing a low-carb diet, Ketogenic diet or intermittent fasting. These types of diets will enable your body to burn the unwanted fats in your body for energy because the supply of carbohydrates is not enough.

When the fats are broken down to produce the energy needed by the body, it releases a type of acid known as ketones that the body can excrete through urine. However, the amount of these ketones should not be too much because it will raise the acidity level in blood. This will cause a condition known as ketoacidosis that is dangerous.

How to Get a Ketosis Process?

Reaching a ketosis state is not something that you can achieve instantly, but it can take you several hours or even days to get to that high fat-burning state. The following are tips that can stimulate your ketosis process.

1. **Reduce Your Carb Intake and Concentrate on Keto Friendly Foods**

Eating a low-carb diet will accelerate your Ketosis. Naturally, your body cells will use glucose and sugars to get energy. However, the body can also get energy from Ketones also known as the fatty acids that the liver converts into energy. Keto-friendly foods are low in carbs and high in healthy fats. You should also include high-quality protein like meat, fish, eggs, and chicken in moderation. Therefore, you should strive at eating 70% fat, 25% protein, and 5% carbs. This kind of meals will help you to stay full for longer.

You should not unless you are feeling hungry. This will ensure that the body keeps very little glucose hence you reach Ketosis faster. You will be feeling so much hunger pangs when starting, but this will reduce once you are on Ketosis. However, if you feel that hunger is too much for you, then eat Keto-friendly foods that are high in fat and have moderate protein. Remember that the portion of your meals should not increase just because you have reduced the carb intake.

You should avoid the following foods that are rich in carbs if you want to get into ketosis:

- Sweetened beverages like sodas, juice, alcoholic beverages.

- Sugary foods like ice cream.

- Starchy vegetables like potatoes, peas, beans, corn.

- Wheat products like bread, pasta, cookies, and doughnuts.

- Cereals like rice, wheat, corn, and their products.

- Unhealthy fats like margarine and corn oil

- Processed foods like canned foods or packaged fast foods.

- Avoid foods that contain preservatives, artificial coloring, and sweeteners.

Here is an example of a Keto meal plan:

Breakfast

· You can have Spinach, eggs, bacon and unsweetened coffee or tea.

Lunch

· You can have vegetable salads, meat, avocado, and broccoli and dress it with olive oil.

Dinner

· You can prepare grilled chicken, zucchini, cauliflower gratin, and some salad dressing.

2. **Increase your physical activity**

Doing physical exercises can help you get rid of stored glycogen in your body. When our bodies get busy in any physical activity, it uses muscle glycogen as a source of energy. Therefore, when the glycogen reserve decreases, the body will resort to burning fat to get the needed energy. Therefore, increasing your physical activities will accelerate your ketosis process.

3. **Try intermittent fasting**

Intermittent fasting is the trending thing for those people who are trying to lose weight. It refers to going for some hours or even days without food. When you do not supply food to your body, it will resort to stored fats to convert it into energy. This will help you in getting rid of unwanted fats in your body hence you will shed some weight in the process. There are several types of intermittent fasting. You can do the 16:8 plan, which means that you will eat within eight hours and then you fast in the remaining 16 hours. You can also go for 24 hours or more without food.

These short and long fasts will put you in a ketosis state. Although most people do intermittent fasting for weight loss, research has shown that it has other health benefits. People suffering from diabetes have found that intermittent fasting decreases blood sugar levels. It also helps in reducing cholesterol and slows down the aging symptoms. As you do the fasting, it is important to listen to your body! If you feel sick or nauseated during the fast, then you should break the fast with some healthy food.

4. **Drink enough water**

We all know that water is life! Water helps in digestion and the removal of toxins from the body system. It is also responsible for transporting important nutrients in the blood cells and other body cells. It also aids the liver in the metabolism process as well as the operations of the kidneys. Therefore, we should always keep our bodies hydrated to enable the proper functioning of the various body organs. Drinking water can also help you in your keto process by preventing the keto side effects like bad breath and dry mouth.

5. **Eat enough protein**

Although we are supposed to eat protein to achieve ketosis, we should not eat an excess of it because the body will convert the excess proteins into fats. Protein should be taken in moderation so that it can help the liver with a supply of amino acids that can be converted into glucose to be used by red blood cells and the brain cells. Proteins will also help you in building muscle mass but excessive of it will alter the production of Ketones in your body.

6. **Watch your electrolyte intake**

When you switch to a low-carb keto diet, the kidneys will get rid of some minerals and water from your system. These minerals are electrolytes and they are magnesium, salts, potassium, and calcium. These minerals are very important in our body system because without them, you will be feeling some fatigue, dizziness, cramps, and mood swings. You can find most of these minerals in the bone broth and some keto-friendly foods. You should use the lite-salt because it has both sodium and potassium in it.

7. **Increase the healthy fat intake**

Eating healthy fats will help you to stay full for longer hence it will prevent unnecessary eating. These fats or oils will help you to reach a ketosis state easily. Some of the healthy fats include:

- Avocado

- Coconut oil

- Olive oil

- Flaxseed

How to Start a Ketosis Process?

1. **Make a plan**

- **Plan keto-friendly meals**

You can make a meal plan for a few days, to begin with. Look for keto meal plans and their recipes online. Some of the most popular keto-friendly foods are eggs, beef, vegetable salads, cucumbers, zucchini, chicken, fish, broccoli, cheese, plain yogurt, mushroom, and cauliflower among others. When preparing these foods, ensure that you use healthy oils like olive oils, coconut oils, and avocado oils.

- **Visit the grocery with the keto-food list**

When going shopping, ensure that you have prepared a keto-friendly shopping list. You can also search online for a keto shopping list to guide you on what to buy. Ensure that you check their labels for information about calories, fat, carb, and protein levels that they contain.

- **Purchase a home testing Ketone kit**

It is good to measure your blood ketone level so that you can know your progress and adjust where appropriate. You can do it with the help of indicator strips or ketone meters. You should do the test at least once daily. If you are on ketosis state, the readings in your ketone testing kit should be between 0.5 mmol/l – 3 mmol/l. You can also check the ketone levels in your blood by testing the blood samples and you can request your doctor to do it.

- **Maintain a ketogenic diet for a week**

After a few days of switching to a keto diet, you may get into a ketosis state. You can then decide on how many days you want to stay on ketosis. However, you should consult your nutritionist or doctor about how long you can safely maintain a ketogenic diet.

2. **Shift to a ketogenic diet**

- **Aim at consuming fewer carbs every day**

You need to reduce your carb intake to less than 50 grams per day. You can achieve this by avoiding high carb foods like pasta, rice, potatoes, wheat products, corn, legumes, and beans. You can replace these foods with low-carb foods.

- **Eat healthy fats**

We mentioned earlier that eating enough healthy fats will keep you feeling full and satisfied for a longer period. Examples of these healthy fat foods include avocados, olive oil, cheese, butter, and coconut oils. You can add these healthy fats into your keto diet to keep you satisfied for longer hours. You can also add whipping cream to your sugarless coffee or tea. Feeling more hunger pangs after switching to a keto diet is an indication that you are not eating enough healthy fats.

- **Avoid starchy vegetables**

The vegetable is very important in our bodies because they carry very essential nutrients however, you should reduce the intake of starchy vegetables so that you can reach ketosis. You should instead eat those vegetables that are very low in carbohydrates like cruciferous vegetables (cabbage, broccoli, cauliflower, and Brussels sprouts), zucchini, cucumbers, spinach, green leaves vegetables, mushroom, and tomatoes.

- **Eat proteins in moderation**

Proteins are very important in a ketogenic diet. However, eating proteins in excess will alter the production of ketones in your body because the body will convert it into glucose. The excess glucose will then be converted and stored as fats. A good source of protein is beef, fish, eggs among others.

- **Include high fiber foods in your diet**

Adding high fiber foods to your diet is important because it aids in digestion. Although most high fiber foods are carbs, you can still find carb-free foods that are high in fiber like flaxseeds, chia seeds, and almonds. Eating high fiber food will help you prevent constipation.

- **Take more coconut oil**

Using extra virgin coconut oil will help you reach your ketosis easily and it comes with other health benefits.

3. **Make lifestyle adjustments**

- **Avoid snacking**

For optimum ketosis state, you should minimize the number of times that you eat in a day. Eating several snacks will hinder you from achieving your ketosis state. You should minimize the snack time you have per day and when you take snacks, ensure that they are keto-friendly. Avoid packaged snacks because most of them contain carbs. You can take low carb snacks like plain yogurt, macadamia nuts or a boiled egg.

- **Drink enough water to stay hydrated**

You need to take enough water every day so that your body organs can function well. You should not drink more than enough water because it will strain the kidneys. Bone broth is also very helpful because it hydrates you as well as provides you with some minerals.

- **Exercise**

When you engage in any physical activity, your body burns carbs into energy and if there is not enough supply of carbs, the body will resort to stored fats for energy. Therefore, exercising can hasten your ketosis process. Exercising for at least 30 minutes daily can give the best results. You can vary your type of exercise to prevent monotony. You can talk a walk, jog around or even run.

- **Get enough sleep**

Getting enough sleep can lower your stress levels. High-stress levels can increase the level of sugar in your blood and this can hinder you from achieving ketosis faster. You should aim at sleeping a minimum of 8 hours daily. This will ensure that your body gets enough rest and re-energizes.

Why Keto Is Convenient

Keto diet is gaining popularity because of its ability to aid in weight loss as well as enhancing the wellbeing of your physical and mental health. The following are some of the reasons why we think keto is convenient.

1. **It helps in weight loss program**

Keto diet is a low carb high-fat diet. Research shows that people who are on a keto diet lose weight faster than those other people who are on a low-fat diet. Since you will be taking high fat and low carb, you will reduce the number of times you eat per day because the high fat and protein will keep you full for longer. The reduction of carbs supply in your body will enable the body to burn stored fats for energy. This will get rid of unwanted fats in your body hence you will shed some weight because of the burned fats.

2. **Reduced blood sugar and insulin levels**

Keto has become very popular among individuals living with diabetes. This is because reducing carbs intake lowers blood sugar and insulin levels and most diabetic people confess that keto has reduced their insulin dosage by a great percentage. Research shows that the keto diet helps in controlling blood sugar and most diabetic patients who are on keto no longer use glucose-lowering medicines. Therefore, reducing carbs intake will give you good blood sugar levels and it can reverse type 2 diabetes. Keto diet has also proven to help in controlling insulin levels in patients with type 1 diabetes.

3. **Helps in treating Epilepsy in children**

A research done in 1998 on 150 children who took carbs restricted diet shows that it was effective in decreasing their seizures by 90%. The keto diet proved to be more helpful on the epilepsy patients more than the anticonvulsant drugs.

4. **Improves blood pressure**

A research done in 2007 showed that a low carb diet was effective in controlling blood pressure. This is because keto diet helps in reducing body mass, LDL cholesterol, and triglycerides. An increase in blood pressure can put you at risk of getting heart diseases and kidney failure. Triglyceride, which is the fat molecules, that circulates in the bloodstream is dangerous because it can cause heart disease.

Reducing carb intake will lower these fat molecules from your bloodstream drastically. On the other hand, LDL is bad cholesterol that circulates in the bloodstream and it can cause heart diseases. Eating a low carb diet will help you to prevent these unpleasant health conditions.

5. Improves the mental Health

Taking too much sugar is not good for your brain and high carbs intake has proved to worsen the condition of Alzheimer patients. Research shows that a keto diet helps to reverse Alzheimer's because the ketone bodies help in improving the memory operations of Alzheimer patients.

Ketone bodies have numerous health benefits to the brain like protecting the brain cells, preserving the neuron, and preventing its loss. Therefore, a low carb diet will significantly improve the health and functions of the brain cells.

6. Helps in the treatment of polycystic ovary syndrome and infertility

Polycystic ovary syndrome (PCOS) is a condition that causes infertility in most women because of the enlarged ovaries that contain cysts. High levels of insulin trigger this condition and it makes the ovaries to release androgens as well as lowering the production of sex hormone. The sex hormone glycoprotein blocks testosterone from getting into the cells. Although there is no such study that shows the relationship between PCOS and diet, keto diet help reduce insulin levels that cause PCOS. Therefore, keto can improve fertility in women.

Testing for Ketosis Process

If you are on a keto diet or fasting, chances are your body is producing ketones. However, you should be in nutritional ketosis where you will reap the most benefits. Therefore, you need to test so that you can know your level of ketosis. Keto diet alone does not determine your level of ketosis. We have other factors like your reaction to food and the activities that you engage in can determine the success of your ketosis.

Testing your ketone levels will help you to understand your progress and adjust your food where necessary. You can adjust your diet and do the testing so that you can know which kinds of food are the most effective in producing more ketones. There are three types of ketone testing:

- The blood tests

- Urine test

- Breath analyzer

The blood test will give the best and most reliable result of the three methods. Our bodies can release three types of ketone bodies namely:

- Acetoacetate: this is the first ketone body that the body produces when there is no longer a supply of glucose for energy. The liver will convert fats into fatty acids, then further converts the fatty acids into ketones. These types of ketones are present in the initial stages of ketosis and it can be detected in urine.

- Acetate (acetone): we get this ketone when acetoacetate is broken down and we exhale it through the lungs as a waste product.

- Beta-hydroxybutyrate (BHB): this is the most common ketone body that is present in blood and goes to cells in the form of energy. It provides the brain cells, muscles, and other body organs with the needed energy.

After reviewing the different types of ketones, we can now look at the various methods that we can use to test ketones in our bodies.

1. **Urine strips**

Urine strips are popular among diabetes patients because they use them to check the diabetes ketones. You can buy urine strips over the counter on any drug store or supermarket pharmacies. You will use it by dipping the strip in the urine collected and wait for a few minutes then read the color of the strip and compare it with the illustrated colors in the package.

The color starts from faint to darker and the darker the strip the more ketones you have in your body.

However, urine strips do not give accurate results. This is because when entering into ketosis, acetoacetate ketones spill into the urine and this might give you a wrong impression on your level of ketosis. The level of hydration in your body will also affect the results of the strip because if you test the urine when you are highly hydrated, the results will not be the same as during dehydration. Therefore, urine strips can only give accurate results for diabetes ketones but not nutritional ketones.

2. Breath test: Acetone indicator

The breath test is for testing acetone, which is a byproduct of breaking down acetoacetate. However, you cannot use it to measure the number of ketones in your body that is working as fuel. You will need a breath meter that you plug into a battery source. You use the breath meter by blowing into it until the flashing light starts reading your breath acetones then you can check the color blinking and the number of times it is blinking then compare with the one illustrated in the package.

There are external factors that can alter the results of the test like chewing gums, cigarettes, toothpaste, garlic, alcohol, and other food substances that can make the sensor malfunction.

Your breathing pace can also affect the acetone level. Therefore, when doing the breath test you need to consider factors like the environment condition, the breathing pace as well as the sensor validity.

You will need to practice breathing techniques severally to get reliable results. You should also purchase a breath meter that allows you to change the sensor and one that you can adjust to a known control.

3. The blood ketone meter

This is the most reliable method of the three. We use the blood ketone meter to measure BHB (beta-hydroxybutyrate) which is the most active ketone body, it circulates in the blood to the cells, and it converts into useful energy. You can do this by taking your blood sample through pricking your finger then squeeze the blood out onto a little strip from the machine and wait for a few seconds to read the machine. Remember to use alcohol to disinfect the area you are pricking to prevent any infection.

There you go; you can now know the BHB level in your blood! You will be able to know the number of ketone bodies that are fueling your body. The advantage of blood ketone meter is that factors like hydration or temperature do not interfere with the outcome unlike in breath tests. Although this method is expensive, it is the best way that you can know your actual ketone levels.

Eliminate the Wrong Convictions of Fat

I grew up with a mentality that fats are not healthy and that I should take a low-fat diet so that I can live a healthy life but I was wrong and I know that I am not alone in this wrong myth. The truth is that there are fats that are good for you and others are bad for your health. Therefore, the belief that a low-fat diet is healthier than a high-fat diet is not justified because it all depends on what kinds of fats you are eating.

There are different types of fats: bad ones and good ones. Monounsaturated fats and polyunsaturated are healthy fats. These fats come from vegetables, nuts, fish, and seeds. The bad fats include the industrial made Trans fats that come in solid kinds of margarine and vegetable shortening while the saturated fats are neither good nor bad and they mostly come from animal products like meat and whole milk.

Our bodies require fats because it helps in absorbing minerals and vitamins. They are also vital in building the cell membranes as well as the sheaths encircling the nerves. The belief that you should eat a low-fat diet to lower your cholesterol is also not true. The following are some of the myths about fats that nutritionist have proven to be wrong.

1. **Eating fat will make you fat**

Eating healthy fats like avocados, olive oil, coconut oil, and butter will help you stay full longer hence; it suppresses your craving for food and the urge to overeat. This can be a useful trick in weight loss management.

2. **Fats are not important in our bodies**

This is not true because healthy fats help us in absorbing important nutrients and vitamins as well as antioxidants and it supplies our bodies with energy. Fats extracted from fish, nuts, and seeds are good for the heart and the brain cells. They also help in weight loss and maintenance. Fats are also responsible for regulating body temperature and hormones.

3. **A low-fat diet is good for weight loss**

This is false. Our bodies require enough fats for energy purposes and the growth of cells. You need to know which good fats are and which ones are not good. Healthy fats like monounsaturated and polyunsaturated fats can be useful in weight loss if you include them in your diets. Most of the packaged foods that write low fat in their label contain sugars. We all know that sugar will hinder weight loss. Other factors can lead to weight gains like excess intake of carbs and calories.

4. **Fats increase cholesterol levels in the bloodstream**

Healthy fats like monounsaturated fats and polyunsaturated fats do not raise the bad cholesterol in your bloodstream but Trans- fats do and you should avoid them. You should also limit the consumption of saturated fats.

5. **Saturated fats clog the arteries**

A research done by a team of cardiologists shows that there is no evidence for this claim because they did not find any relationship between the consumption of saturated fats and the risk of heart diseases. They instead said that people should eat healthy food and exercise to prevent coronary diseases instead of blaming it on the dietary saturated fats. They also noted that patients living with chronic inflammatory disease responded well with eating healthy fats like olive oil, and the oils from nuts and fish. The omega 3 fatty acids found in these oils helps in preventing heart diseases.

Take away

It is important to know what kind of fat you are consuming because healthy fats are very crucial for healthy living while Trans fats can cause problems for your health.

Control Calories with Low Carb

Calories refer to the amount of energy that you get from food and the energy you use on physical activities. For weight gain, you subtract the calorie going out from the calorie coming in. If you want to lose weight then you should control your calorie intake even if you are on a keto diet or you can increase your physical activities so that you can burn the excess calories. The number of calories that you can consume will depend on what you want to achieve, how physically active you are and your basal metabolic rate (BMR).

Eating a low carb diet can generally reduce the number of calories that you consume because the macronutrients from high fat, protein, and low carb suppress the cravings for food. However, if you take the high-fat diet in excess, it can add up to more calorie intake. Most of the Keto-friendly foods like avocados, olive oil, and full-fat dairy contain a high amount of calories so you should eat them in moderation if you plan to lose weight.

To control the calories in a keto diet, you need to be very meticulous when it comes to your food portion. You also need to consider engaging in physical exercises to ensure that you burn more calories than the amount you take. If your plan is just to reach ketosis and improve your well-being, then your attention should be on the quality of the food you eat and not calories. However, if your main aim is to cut some weight, then you will need to watch your calorie intake and adjust appropriately.

You may not alter the amount of protein and carbs you take while on keto but you can adjust the amounts of fat so that you can monitor the caloric intake. The carb levels should be low and you can focus on the green leafy vegetables while you eat proteins in moderation to help you in building your mass muscles.

Therefore, it is important to track the number of calories that you take as well as the macronutrient's quality. This will ensure that you do not experience some nutrient deficiencies as well as gain weight from consuming too many calories. On the other hand, you should engage in physical exercises to keep you fit.

Keto Health

Keto diet is among the trending diet plans available. It is popular among diabetic patients and those people who wish to lose weight. It involves taking 75% high-fat food, 20% protein, and only 5% carbs. After a few days of observing this percentage of foods in your diet, your body will get into a state called ketosis whereby the body burns stored fat in the body. Therefore, this diet plan restricts carb intake and focuses on taking a high-fat diet.

The following are some health benefits of keto:

1. **Helps in weight loss**

Perhaps this is the #1 reason why keto gained popularity. Keto helps in burning stored fats and suppressing the cravings for food so this will prevent frequent snacking. Eating fewer carbs also will help in reducing the amount of calorie intake and the protein and fat in the diet will provide a satiating effect.

When carbs intake reduces, the body's metabolism changes and accelerates the burning of fat to get energy. Therefore, the body uses most of the fat sources and converts it into energy. This process of burning fat will enable the body to burn calories too. However, to get rid of more calories you need to ensure that you limit the calorie intake and do more activities that are physical.

2. **Blood sugar control**

Keto helps in stabilizing blood sugar and the mood swings that come with the fluctuation of blood sugar levels. Keto diet is helpful to diabetes patients because the low carb intake prevents the huge spikes in blood sugar hence lowering the need for insulin. However, you should be careful not to combine a keto diet with insulin because it can lead to hypoglycemia a condition for low blood sugar. Ensure that you talk with your doctor concerning your switch of diet while on medication.

3. **Keto improves brain function and mental health**

Ketosis helps in protecting the brain from damage by shifting the energy source and regulating the energy metabolism genes. It also protects it from oxidative stress that can damage it. Oxidative stress promotes brain aging, depression, and anxiety. Ketones provide the brain with energy when it cannot get it from glucose and this helps to improve memory performance by balancing the brain chemicals.

People doing keto confess that it provides them with mental sharpness and creativity that helps them to handle multitasking while they maintain a motivated attitude. It increases blood flow to the brain hence reinforcing the various memory and sensory operations. Keto can treat epilepsy in children because of its ability to reconnect brain energy metabolism. Epileptic kids who shift to keto decrease their seizure by a greater percentage.

4. **Eliminates food cravings**

Eating a high fat, moderate protein, and low carb diet will give you a satiating effect. It will make you feel full for longer hence your appetite for frequent snacking will no longer be there. This will help you to focus on eating healthy low carb diets during the main meals. You will no longer have to worry about your addiction to overeating because keto will put your appetite under control.

5. **Reduces anxiety and depression**

Keto helps protect the brain from the damage of oxidative stress that can cause depression and anxiety. Keto diet stabilizes blood sugar that can cause fluctuation in mood swings. Therefore, being on keto can keep your moods on track!

6. **Good for your heart**

Keto can help you to lose weight that can lead to cardiovascular diseases such as high blood pressure, high blood sugar that can cause the inflammation of the arteries and increase in bad cholesterol. These conditions are not good for the heart. Therefore, keto helps in preventing the conditions that can be harmful to the heart.

The Downside of Keto

Although you can reap many benefits from a keto diet, there is an unpleasant downside of this diet plan and you should study it carefully if you plan to do it on a long-term basis. Some of the side effects occur naturally while you are on keto while others can occur if you do it the wrong way. The medical community, however, points out that keto might not be a safe long-term diet plan. Here are some of the unpleasant downsides that you will experience while on keto.

1. **Keto flu**

During the first weeks of being on keto, your body will be struggling to adapt to the new diet and the carb reduction. As a result, you will lose some water and electrolytes and this might make you feel sick. The keto flu symptoms are:

- Frequent headaches

- Fatigue

- Nausea

- Dizziness

- Brain fog

- Irritability

These symptoms can subsidize when your body enters ketosis state. You will need to press on until your body gets used to a low supply of carbohydrates.

2. **Nutritional deficiencies**

Keto diet is a restricted diet. That means there are some foods that you are not supposed to eat while on keto. The foods that you restrict or ban from your diet contain some essential nutrients to your well-being. Beans, legumes, fruits, and some vegetables provide us with vitamin C and fiber yet keto restricts its intake. Therefore, keto will deprive you of getting very important nutrients by eliminating certain food from your diet.

3. **Limited food choice**

Keto involves restriction of carbs yet most of the foods available contain carbs. If you are restricting carb intake, then it means that you will have a list of foods to choose from in your diet. You will need to cut off all the grains and their products as well as all the starchy vegetables and all the sugars. This diet plan may not be sustainable in the end because you will be craving for foods that you eliminated.

4. **Expensive**

Most of the keto meal plans are expensive compared to non-keto meals. The oils used in the keto diet like olive oils, coconut oils, and fish oils are also quite expensive when you compare to the ordinary cooking oils. You can find avocados when they are in season but the avocado oil can be hard to find not to mention its high cost.

5. **Loss of electrolytes**

When your body reaches a ketosis state, it will start eliminating glycogen from the muscles and the liver and this can lead to frequent urination. When you lose more water in your body, you also lose electrolytes like sodium, potassium, and magnesium that are very crucial for heart operations.

Therefore, you will have to look for electrolyte supplements to replace the lost ones.

6. Health concerns

There is no existing study on the long-term safety of keto use but the medical community suggests that long-term use may not be healthy. People who have used keto for long reported digestion problems like constipation, diarrhea, and bloating. Lack of enough fiber in the diet is the main reason for such stomach problems.

Kidney stones are another common problem for someone who uses a keto diet for several months or even years. People reported to having abdominal pains that later turned to be kidney stones. This could be the effects of consuming too much animal proteins.

Ketoacidosis is also a problem that can occur while you are on a keto diet. This occurs when the body produces too much ketone bodies and the blood become too acidic. This condition is dangerous because it can damage the kidneys, liver and even the brain. Ketoacidosis can affect most people with diabetes and are on a keto diet. Therefore, diabetic individuals need to be extra watchful of their glucose levels while on keto.

Patients suffering from liver failure, pancreatitis, a disorder of fat metabolism, should consult their doctors before getting into keto. Although keto helps improve fertility in women, research shows that it can harm the growing fetus because it will lack some important nutrients that are crucial for its growth and development. You also need to check your body regularly if you have a history of anemia in your family. This is because a nutritional deficiency can put you at risk of contracting it.

7. **Weakened immune system**

Eating high fat and less fiber can mess with the balance of good and bad bacteria in your gastrointestinal tract. Since the GI protects your immune system, the imbalance of bacteria in it can have an impact on the gut-brain connection as well as the immune connection and this can cause diseases.

Fruits and vegetables are good for protecting the immune system. However, keto restricts the intake of vegetables and fruits that contains carbs this can make you susceptible to chronic illness or long-term diseases.

Keto for Weight Loss

Keto diet is high in healthy fat with moderate protein and low carbs. Since your body will cut down the supply of carbs that is supposed to provide glucose for energy, the body will source for glucose elsewhere within the body. The liver can rescue your body with energy by converting the stored fats into ketone bodies. This process is ketosis.

To reach ketosis, you will need to restrict your daily carb intake to less than 50 grams. If you aim to lose weight, then you have to watch the calories you consume through fats. You also have to ensure that the fats that you consume are healthy ones like olive oil, avocado oils, and nuts. Remember that it is important to engage in physical exercises so that your body can burn excess calories.

Keto is a great tool for weight loss because the high fat and the protein in the diet will keep you feeling full for longer hence you will reduce the number of snack times as well as the calorie intake. Keto will help you to suppress your appetite for food giving you more self-control on what you can eat. It will also supply you with the needed energy for physical activities. Therefore, the keto diet is good enough for those people who wish to cut some weight.

Chapter 3: Ways to Start the Keto Lifestyle

Past Perspective on Your Diet

Food is generally supposed to be eaten to provide nourishment to the body. It is the source of energy as well as the fuel for growth. Human beings eat food for a number of reasons. They can eat to celebrate a certain occasion while they make merry with friends and family. They also eat for pleasure especially when they are socializing. Sometimes, people eat because they have nothing else to do, they can do so out of boredom or loneliness. Food can also be consumed out of habit or because a person is accustomed to certain traditions.

A good number of people turn to food when they are stressed or anxious about something. Food in such cases becomes a drug for comfort. Rather than turn to habits such as drinking or smoking these kinds of people get their high from food. Notably, just as with the case of drunks and smokers, emotional eaters also regret their choices soon after they indulge in an unhealthy meal. Eventually, they also suffer the consequences of their 'substance abuse'.

People's intake of food also depends on an individual's lifestyle. For example, there are those people who like staying fit so they are very cautious about what they put in their mouths. They also exercise on a regular basis to keep their weight on check. Although they may appear to be healthy, some of them struggle to maintain their lifestyle. They agonize over what they are missing out, how to avoid social gatherings or people who may mislead them from their diet plans. Spending too much time planning for the next meal in addition to the agony of wanting to burn off excess calories after indulging in a treat eventually begins to stress them out.

For another set of people, their lives are too chaotic for them to sit and have a decent meal. A working mom, for example, who juggles a hectic work schedule, family time and volunteer work, might not find time to eat healthily. She may result in eating while on the move or multitask while eating. This means that she eats while driving or walking to a meeting or when answering phone calls and emails. This mom will only eat a proper meal when she gets back to the house. If she is too tired to eat, she will have another snack and retire to bed. She may also want to eat healthily and is clearly aware that she should eat more nutritional food but is unable to do so because of her crazy work schedule.

There is also another group of people who seem to be unaffected by what they eat. They are not bothered by what they eat nor do they care to follow diets or engage in exercise. Those who manage to remain slender after all the eating is the envy of many. A majority of natural eaters, however, appear soft and round. Some may appear strong and built because of either their genes or engaging in some form of physical activity that builds muscle.

Wherever you fall in the above categories, you should always ensure that your diet has the right amount of calories. A proper diet should not too little calories or too many calories. The exercise junky might be getting too few calories while the natural eater might be consuming too many calories. People who do not get enough calories end up losing muscle mass and succumb to health problems. Eating too many calories leads to high blood pressure, heart disease, diabetes or even death.

A healthy diet should also have the right amounts of fat and the right type of fat. Generally, it is advisable to avoid unhealthy fats such as saturated fats found in fatty meat and dairy products such as butter and cream. Trans-fats found in commercial foods such as cakes and fried junk food should be kept to a minimal. Fats increase cholesterol levels in the blood and can block arteries or cause heart attacks and stroke.

High amounts of sugar in a diet also put you at risk of gaining weight and developing health problems similar to the ones listed above. Sugar comes in many forms and therefore has different names. Added sugar is a very common ingredient in modern diets and people should avoid anything that has added sugar. High consumption of sugar leads to weight gain and is associated with diseases such as type 2 diabetes and heart disease.

Fruits and vegetables should be consumed in large amounts but they seem to make the least appearance in most people's diets. People are also choosing to substitute water with other unhealthy drinks that are harmful to the body. Salt is also consumed but sometimes at extreme levels while nuts and seeds are not incorporated on a regular basis.

In an attempt to overcome unhealthy eating habits people also get into all sorts of diets. Fad diets are unrealistic and as much as they may help a person lose weight on the onset, most are not sustainable. They also deprive people of healthy foods that are important to the body. Any person who wants to start a diet allows them to consume foods from most if not all food groups but of course, everything should be consumed in moderation. Exercise is also important in maintaining a healthy weight and general health of the body.

It is important to review your diet and reason out whether the diet you are following offers the right amounts of nutrients that are able to feed and nourish your cells as well as give you a general feeling of happiness. A good diet should also enable you to eliminate waste on a regular basis and give you energy.

Wrong Eating Habits

Most people have an idea of what they should and should not eat. Some have even gone a step further to carefully plan their meals and sign up for fitness classes. However, for some reason, they are still not able to achieve healthy weight levels. Healthy eating does not just involve eating the right types of foods; how people eat and the habits they form around food contribute a great deal, to whether or not they live happy and healthy lifestyles.

The number one cause of unhealthy diets is, of course, unhealthy food. Foods that contain high amounts of fat, calories, and sugar are considered unhealthy. The quality of food that you put in your mouth matters and affects your health. The best diets include foods from every group. They also include both animal and plant sources. Eating unhealthy fats raises your cholesterol levels so does eating excess carbohydrates and proteins. Occasionally, you can indulge in your favorite snack but you should remember to do it in moderation. Other healthy foods such as vegetables, fruits, and nuts are eaten in minimal quantities when they should occupy the most amount of space on your plate.

Some wrong eating habits that people have gotten accustomed to include:

1. Stocking up on tempting snacks

It is very hard to keep away from the food that you can see and is within your reach. Sometimes even storing unhealthy snacks inside the cupboard or just in the house can tempt you to eat them. It is best to avoid stacking snacks in the house. If you have to snack keep fresh pre-chopped vegetables and fruits on the countertop.

2. Skipping breakfast

Breakfast is the most important meal of the day. When you load on a healthy breakfast, you get enough energy to take on the day. When you skip it, your metabolism slows down and you increase your chances of binging on an unhealthy snack or meal later on in the day because you are too hungry. Skipping breakfast eventually leads to weight gain in the end. Rushing through breakfast is also not advised.

3. Mindless eating

Mindless eating or snacking leads to unhealthy weight gain and it occurs when a TV, video game, or working on a computer, distracts people. Binging in front of the TV makes you gain weight in two ways. Eating while distracted by something else makes you eat more. You unknowingly consume larger portions of food especially if you are eating from a large bowl or out of a box. Most of the time when you eat out of a bag, you normally eat more than one serving, even several without knowing. This contributes to weight gain. If you have a habit of sitting or lying down for long hours, physical inactivity can make you retain a lot of weight.

4. Midnight and endless snacking

Eating at night is never a good idea. When people eat dinner and then go to bed immediately, their food does not get digested properly. When you also snack in the middle of the night, you also do not give the food time to digest well. Sleeping also puts the body in a state of inactivity meaning that the food consumed does not burn to energy so it has to be stored in the body and this contributes to weight gain. The other problem with midnight snacking is the fact that people rarely snack on healthy foods. Most commercial snacks are unhealthy, they are either high in unhealthy fats, calories or contain added sugar and high amounts of salt. Unhealthy snacking during the day is also not advisable.

5. Eating on the move

When you eat while driving or walking in most cases, you are not conscious of how much you are putting in your mouth, so you end up eating a lot of food. The other activity you are engaged in also acts as a distraction so you end up consuming more food unknowingly. The other challenge with eating while distracted with another activity and eating quickly for that matter is that you do not give your body enough time to register that you are full. Your brain takes time to receive the message that you are full and needs time to signal to you that you should stop eating. When you eat slowly and chew your food the right away, you give your body organs time to communicate with one another. Even the simple act of putting the spoon down or taking a sip of water slows you down to think whether you are full or not.

6. Eat out or order in too much

Most foods prepared in restaurants and fast foods are not prepared with healthy eating in mind. These foods are prepared to fulfill taste and flavor rather than nutrition. Restaurant meals are also normally served with extra sauces drizzled with excess oil and the quantities are usually more. It is very easy to gain weight when you constantly eat out or order in food. Most takeout meals or foods that are delivered are normally junk food, such as burgers, fries, or pizzas. Unlike when food is prepared at home, you also do not have much control over what unhealthy food items or spices are put in your food.

7. Take unhealthy drinks

Your favorite latte in the morning or cappuccino could just be as unhealthy as eating junk food and so is downing a flavored drink. It is very possible to consume more calories from a drink than a meal. In addition to the calories, some drinks contain high levels of sugar and the frothy drinks contain unhealthy fats. These drinks also replace water intake, which is very crucial in maintaining good health. Alcoholic drinks, on the other hand, add to the calories you consume.

Wrong Food Combinations

All health experts condone overindulging in unhealthy meals. Most people are aware of the health risks and dangers associated with consuming unhealthy meals. Healthy meals that are combined in the wrong way are at times just as harmful as eating unhealthy meals.

1. Carbs and animal protein

A combination of steak and fries is bad. The starch in potatoes normally requires alkaline juices to digest while proteins require an acidic environment to be broken down. When the two are eaten together, they remain in the stomach and bring discomforts such as gas, flatulence, and heartburn. The same goes for a combination such as pasta and minced meat. The starch in pasta is converted to sugar and when combined with the meat, a person can develop diabetes. With time, a person who eats such combinations develops immunity but the excess intake, especially with a combination of fatty oils from both foods, leads to elevated cholesterol levels and unhealthy weight gain. It is okay to combine carbs with healthy plant protein such as beans that is why a combination such as rice and beans is not only delicious but also yummy.

2. Two high proteins

People are notorious for eating more than one protein and heavy ones for that matter during breakfast. One of the most popular combinations is bacon and eggs. As much as a person remains full for longer, the combination overworks the digestive system. This combination also gives a high-energy boost immediately after the meal but it also disappears after a short denying you proper energy to begin the day. Two proteins also take longer to digest. When you eat two proteins at the same time, it is advisable that you combine a light protein and heavy one but not two heavy proteins. The lighter one should be eaten first followed by the heavy one and the two should not be spaced out too much. They should also be eaten within 10 minutes of each other. A combination such as beans and cheese also fall in this category of two high proteins. They are both heavy to digest. Cheese and meat are also two high proteins that are difficult to digest.

3. Food with drinks

Food should never be taken with any beverage, even water. Water normally dilutes stomach acids, which digest food. It reduces the ability of the acid to breakdown the food in the stomach. Water or juices took immediately after meals also have the same effects on the digestive system.

4. Fruits after meals

We all love to fish with a juicy mango salad but experts advise that this is another disastrous food combination that people should avoid. Essentially fruits should be eaten before meals as they pass through the digestive system faster. When they are combined with a meal and especially a heavy protein, they have to stay in the digestive tract for long and the sugar in them begins to ferment. You may think that you are making a healthy food choice when you eat fruit instead of a slice of cake after a meal but you are also not doing the right thing for your body. If you have to eat fruit with a meal, it is always good to eat it before the meal.

5. Yogurt with fruit

Most of us have eaten this combination without giving it a second thought; both items are healthy with the yogurt providing a good dose of protein and calcium as well as good bacteria and the fruits bursting with vitamins. However, the two together are a bad idea. Milk and acid generally do not mix well. Since fruits are acidic, they are never a good fit for yogurt. The bacterium in yogurt also likes the sugar in fruit and does not hesitate to act on it. Dairy is also known for causing sinuses and cold allergies when it is combined with fruit, its effects worsen.

6.   Cereal with juice

Cereal is a popular food item during breakfast and it normally goes well with milk. There are people who add juice to this combination, however, as earlier deduced the acid in juice is never a good combination with dairy products. The casein in milk and the acid together, normally curdle milk. The combination also destroys enzymes found in the starch of the cereal. The carbohydrate in cereal is therefore not broken down well. The discomfort after eating this combination is characterized by a feeling of heaviness.

7.   Tomatoes with pasta

Although this is a favorite among many people, the combination causes havoc in the stomach. Worse still is when the meal is combined with cheese. The acid in tomatoes curdles the dairy in cheese and interferes with the enzymes that digest starch in the pasta. Meats and carbs as earlier stated are also not one of the best combinations of foods.

8.   Milk with banana

This is another popular combination probably because it is very easy to prepare. The sugar in the banana also adds a sweet taste to the milk. Banana is a fruit and like many fruits, it should not be consumed with dairy products. When fruits and especially sweet ones are combined with other foods, milk included, they stay in the digestive system for longer. Rather than add fruits to milk, a pinch of nutmeg or cinnamon stimulates the digestive system and does not slow it down.

Healthy Keto Food Combinations

The keto diet is becoming popular. However, a number of people are still not been able to achieve any substantial results with it. If people are not keen on both how and what they eat and the combinations of food that they eat, then they can hardly sustain the diets that they are following.

A proper keto diet should be high in healthy fats, it should have moderate amounts of protein and carbohydrates should be low. The fact that a keto diet helps you get rid of carbohydrates and bulks you on protein and starch should not be a reason for you to stock up on bacon and burgers. Although there is nothing wrong with a little bacon and butter, most of the food in the keto diet should be plant-based and then the protein and fat can be added on top of greens.

Vegetables provide healthy carbohydrates as well as fiber. Insoluble fiber cannot be broken down by bacteria neither does it dissolve in water. This means that it stays in the gut and cleans it up. It also helps the gut retain a lot of water, which makes waste softer and enables it to pass through easily.

Keto diets should also have resistant starches, which keep you fuller for longer. Some foods that have resistant starch in abundance include legumes, bananas, peas, and oats. Eating these types of foods prevent you from overeating proteins and carbohydrates. Aside from suppressing hunger, they also do not elevate blood glucose levels, unlike excess protein and carbs. Excess protein raises insulin levels the same way carbohydrates do. It is normally converted to glucose and stored as fat in the body.

Therefore, as you think of starting or resuming a keto diet, you should keep in mind that plants should take up more space followed by fats and then protein. Here are some good keto combinations

1. Vegetables drizzled with oil

Low carb vegetables such as broccoli, mushroom, celery, kale, or peppers are good choices in a keto diet. Pouring a generous amount of healthy oil such as olive oil on top of the vegetable makes a good keto meal. Ghee can also be used in place of the olive oil. Coconut oil can also make a great substitute. Since ketogenic diets also allow for moderate amounts of protein, cheese sprinkles can be added to the vegetables to provide nutrition and flavor. Unhealthy oils such as margarine should be avoided. Shortening oils and vegetable oils are also not healthy compared to super oils such as coconut and olive oils. You can prepare a combination of vegetables as long as you keep carbs on the check.

2. Chicken and avocado

Chicken is a very good source of protein while avocado is a good source of healthy fat, which makes this combination perfect for a person following the keto diet. Chicken can also be prepared in very many ways and according to a person's taste. Its diversity also ensures that a person is able to eat this meal in different ways, which means that they do not easily get bored with it. The chicken can be boiled, grilled, or roasted and can be substituted with fish to make a healthy complete keto meal. Turkey can also be used in place of the chicken.

3. Fish and sour cream

If the taste of fish with avocado does not tingle your taste buds, you can try fish with some sour cream. A number of people like their fish with a slice of lemon but this would not make a complete keto meal. It lacks a vegetable and healthy fat. Fish is rich in protein and in addition to being a good source of protein, fish also has omega 3 which are healthy for the brain. The sour cream, on the other hand, brings in fat, which is essential in a keto diet. It also enhances the flavor of the fish. You can also ditch the sour cream altogether and have a grilled salmon combined with sautéed vegetables. Coconut oil can be used to sauté a good serving of spinach.

4. **Pork chops with green beans**

This combination can be eaten for dinner and is very filling. The pork, of course, provides the protein while the green beans sautéed in healthy oil such as coconut oil bring in the element of fat and vegetable nutrition.

5. **Eggs and cheese**

If you are looking for something healthy to have for breakfast while on a keto diet, eggs and cheese are a healthy combination. Rather than have eggs and bacon which are two high proteins, eggs and cheese is a much healthier combination. The egg provides the protein while the cheese provides an excellent source of fat. Cheese also contains protein but when combined with eggs, the protein intake is not too high as with other combinations such as meat and cheese. Eggs and cheese can also be used together in a Cobb salad. In addition to these two ingredients, a Cobb salad can have slices of turkey and a green vegetable especially one that is low on carbs. You can also substitute the cheese and use a plant protein such as a mushroom; these two food items together with a bit of oil can make a tasty mushroom omelet. Eggs served with sautéed greens can also provide a healthy keto breakfast.

6. Healthy keto smoothies

Yogurt and fruits are not a good combination as earlier stated but yogurt and nuts go very well together. Greek yogurt enriched with nuts such as almonds, cashews or walnuts is a very healthy snack perfect for anyone on a keto diet. Yogurt is dairy and therefore provides a good dose of protein. It also has friendly bacteria that are good for your gut. Since regular dairy milk is not healthy if combined with fruits, an avocado can be combined with coconut milk to produce healthy coconut milk and avocado smoothie.

Water is very important in any diet and more so in a keto diet that is low in carbs. Carbs not only provide energy for the body but they also help the body to retain water. Any extra carbs are normally stored as glycogen in the liver. For the glycogen to stay together it needs water. Since ketogenic diets are low on carbs, there are normally no extra carbs to store in the liver, which means that the water molecules are also not needed. Therefore, a person on any low carb diet should ensure that they drink a lot of water, even more than the recommended eight glasses of water. Most alcoholic drinks and sweet drinks should be avoided mainly because they add carbs to the die. To have a variety of beverages, you can flavor your water or take sparkling water in place of soda. If you enjoy coffee and tea, you should keep it as plain as possible and avoid adding sugar.

Of course, electrolytes which include sodium, potassium, and magnesium should also be present in any diet include a keto diet. It is very easy to lose these minerals because of the way the diet flashes out water from the body. To avoid this, a person on a low carb diet can consciously add salt or take supplements, otherwise, they risk contracting what is commonly known as the keto flu.

Chapter 4: Keto Shopping List

What healthy options should you consider having in your grocery-shopping list? Spinach and arugula, avocados, cucumbers, berries, olive oil, almond butter, parmesan and gouda cheese, natural yogurt, lamb chops, chicken, turkey, tuna, salmon, sardines, cod, bacon, walnuts, chia seeds, and flax seeds.

Keto is a high fat, high-protein, and low-carb eating plan that enables a person's body to burn fat instead of carbs for fuel, and ultimately leading to substantial weight loss.

The human body breaks down, carbohydrates into glucose, which the body uses for energy. When the body does not have enough energy, it goes into a state called Ketosis. During ketosis, the body burns fat and uses it for energy, in place of the glucose.

Ketosis, therefore, makes the ketogenic diet a popular option for people who want to lose weight. However, a person's body needs to go into ketosis before a person can begin to lose weight on the keto diet. That means reducing the intake of carbohydrates to the minimum. A diet that provides fewer than 50 grams of carbs per day can cause ketosis.

Keto Supplements

Certain supplements help to support a person's immune system and prevent nutrient deficiencies.

Here are the best supplements to consider having in your keto diet.

1. **Plant-based MCT oil**: Medium-Chain-Triglycerides (MCT) comes from coconut or palm oil. A person can put a tablespoon or two to a coffee or a smoothie to reach ketosis and improve mental energy.

    MCT oil gives high levels of circulating ketones in the blood, which fuels the brain cells and curb a person's appetite. A person should start with small doses to avoid stomach pain.

2. **Omega-3 fatty acids**: Fish oils are a valuable source of heart-healthy omega 3- fatty acids. The fats are essential for reducing cholesterol numbers connected to cardiovascular disease.

    Exposure to plant oils and clean sources of fish oils increases the chances of lowering cholesterol levels in a person's body.

3. **Magnesium supplements**: Magnesium is an essential nutrient for muscle and bone health and regulation of blood pressure. However, magnesium-

rich foods like fruits and beans are high in carbs and can kick a person out of ketosis.

Therefore, a person can substitute such foods for foods such as avocados and spinach that are low on magnesium.

4. **BHB Salts**: Beta-hydroxybutyrate (BHB) is an energy particle that a person's body produces when breaking down and burning fat. When a person is in ketosis, he or she has higher levels of BHB.

   BHB salts facilitate a person's brain to lower the production of glucose and turn to burn fat instead.

5. **Collagen supplements**: Collagen is an animal protein that comes from the bones, bone marrows and the connective tissues of the animal.

   Collagen is a high source of energy that helps to strengthen muscles because ketosis can feed on the muscle if a person does not have enough fat for fuel. Collagen supplements have to contain MCT oil powder to make it keto-friendly.

6. **Calcium supplements**: Cheese, yogurt, and milk are rich in calcium but also high in carbs. Therefore, a person has to reduce the intake of such calcium-rich foods to minimize carbs.

Alternatively, a person can obtain calcium from sardines, salmon, and mackerel with edible bones. In addition, the person can get calcium from calcium citrate or calcium carbonate supplements, which he or she should eat, with food to ensure maximum absorption.

7. **Digestive enzymes**: Digestive enzymes break down fats and proteins to facilitate a person's digestion and to prevent constipation.

   Fatty foods can increase chances of constipation, but digestive enzymes have lipase and protease that help to improve a person's digestion, in the absence of fiber-rich carbohydrates.

8. **Fiber supplements**: Fiber supplements such as psyllium increase fiber in ketogenic diets. A person should allow time for his or her gastrointestinal (GI) tract to adapt to the high fiber intake, to avoid cramping and gas.

   Other keto-friendly fiber sources include cauliflower and brussels sprouts.

9. **Multivitamins Supplements**: Multivitamin keto supplements help to keep a person's body functioning normally by supplying the specific nutrients level that the body needs.

A person can take multivitamins that provide the B vitamins, to make up for his or her reduced intake of whole grains and legumes.

10. **Vitamin B complex supplements**: Vitamin B supplements help to reduce exhaustion, cramping, and brain fog. These are the symptoms a person experiences when switching to a low-carb eating plan.

   Vitamin B increases blood sugar and brain energy levels as fats replace carbs as the body's primary source of energy.

11. **Electrolyte supplements**: Electrolyte supplements help to replace the levels of sodium, magnesium, and potassium that a person loses when taking the keto diet.

   A person can begin to cut off water weight when the level of electrolytes goes down. A person loses great amounts of fluid through the keto diet, but the electrolyte supplements help to prevent such loss of electrolytes.

12. **Vitamin D3 supplements**: Vitamin D3 is essential for helping a person's body to absorb calcium. In that way, Vitamin D3 boosts the growth of body cells, reduces inflammation, and maintains the health of a person's bones.

Alternatively, a person can get this sunshine vitamin by exposing himself or herself to the sunrays. However, that exposure may not be enough to help a person's body to produce Vitamin D naturally.

Hormones Balance in Keto

A ketogenic diet helps to regulate specific hormone imbalances naturally. Here are ways in which going keto helps to put a person's body back in order.

1. Keto diet cools hot flashes

High estrogen levels cause the part of the brain that controls stress to become unstable when prompted abruptly. As a result, the body's temperature increases and then decreases within minutes.

Keto diet supplies the body with a continuous source of fuel, ketones, for the brain. In so doing, the hot flashes cool down. Hot flashes make menopausal women and those with Polycystic ovary syndrome (PCOS) to have distressing periods of a sudden rise in their body temperature.

2. Keto diet decreases inflammations

Inflammation can be good when it is an immune response to protect the body from disease and infection, and harmful when it causes inflammatory disorders.

Studies show that low-carb diets reduce the chances of inflammation by a more considerable margin than consuming low-fat diets. Ketogenic diets prevent factors responsible for chronic inflammation by activating a complex biochemical process that fights inflammation directly.

In addition, biochemical activity helps to reduce chronic inflammations related to health problems.

3. Keto diet facilitates weight loss

Since keto can regulate ghrelin and leptin, the hormones that bring an appetite, therefore a person following a keto diet can feel less hungry.

When ghrelin and leptin are not balanced, a person usually feels always hungry even when he or she eats something. The irregular increase in levels of hunger and decrease in fullness after eating prompts a person's craving to ingest more glucose.

Because the keto diet helps to balance these hormones, a person on a keto diet will, therefore, eat less and lose weight more naturally.

4. Keto diet increases energy levels

High energy levels during the day help people to sleep better at night. That is because keto helps to control levels of cortisol in the body, thus reducing stress levels and increasing energy production.

Keto diets provide slower-burning forms of energy that regulate blood sugar levels and produce enough energy for the day. Hormonal imbalance can increase the levels of cortisol production in the body. The stress hormone can suck up a person's energy and bring about restless sleep.

5. Keto diet lowers blood pressure

A ketogenic diet lowers blood pressure by helping in weight loss. Being overweight is one of the top causes of high blood pressure.

A keto diet that takes processed foods off the shopping list, promotes foods that lower high levels of blood sugar in a person's body and reduces cholesterol levels and blood pressure.

High blood pressure is a risk feature for cardiovascular disease and can harm the well-being of a person's heart.

6. Promotes mental health

Hormonal imbalance can affect brain activity negatively. That is because the imbalance can reduce brain function.

Such cognitive glitches come about because of the brain's need for fuel. The brain struggles to get fuel when there is low production of hormones. However, the keto diet provides alternative sources of fuel that regulate energy stability in the body.

When a person has stable energy levels, hormones regain balance and thus improve the cognitive function.

Keto Aliments Can Kill Cancer

Although no single food can cure disease, research shows that the keto diet shows some degree of potential in reducing the growth of certain tumors. That includes slowing the growth of tumors, prolonging the survival rate of cancer patients, and delaying the initial growth stages of tumors.

Keto aliments improve the effectiveness of standard chemotherapy because the diet helps to keep the blood sugar in check. Cancer patients can benefit from the ketogenic diet by following the diet, along with their chemotherapy or cancer treatments.

Chemotherapy and cancer treatments are much more effective when a cancer patient takes in low-carb meals. Health practitioners recommend patients to eat 70 to 80 percent fat, and 10 to 25 percent protein to help with cancer treatment. However, health experts do not guarantee that the keto diet can help to prevent cancer.

Keto diet strengthens regular cancer treatment by inducing metabolic oxidative stress in cancer cells, but not in the healthy cells. In addition, some cancer cells rely heavily on glucose for energy. Therefore, limiting the access of cancer cells to glucose may cause the cancer cells to respond positively to chemotherapy.

According to research, the keto diet, along with the medical restriction of blood glucose prevents the growth of squamous cell carcinoma (SCC) in mice with lung cancer. Even though such interventions did not reduce the size of the tumors in the mice, they prevented the tumors from developing. That only applied to the SCC cancers and not to the lung adenocarcinoma cancers.

However, it is still too early to tell whether the outcomes of the research can apply to humans. For now, the keto diet may only act as a complementary therapy for some patients going through cancer treatment.

That is to say that when cancer patients follow a ketogenic diet, they help to strengthen their metabolic network systems throughout the body. As long as a person's mitochondria stay healthy and useful, it is very unlikely that the person will develop cancer.

In the meantime, health specialists will continue to carry out more comprehensive and detailed clinical studies on the subject.

Keto Aliments for Brain Health

Keto diets provide energy to the brain through a process called ketogenesis. Glucose is the primary source of energy for the brain, and the brain cannot use fat as a source of energy.

However, the brain can use ketones that the liver produces when the level of glucose and insulin in a person's body is low. When a person eliminates carbs from his or her diet, ketones can give up to 70 percent of the brain's energy. However, that means that the body is still getting 20 to 25 percent of its energy from glucose.

Therefore, even when a person is in ketosis, his or her body is still finding a way to generate blood sugar and have glucose in the system. The brain will always have glucose demands. Similarly, a person will eliminate glucose from his or her body.

A ketogenic diet helps to multiply the number of mitochondria in the brain cells, which helps to improve mild cognitive impairment and memory scores. Ketones elicit more response than glucose does inside the mitochondria. That is because there is more energy per unit of oxygen combined with the ketone than there is energy created when oxygen combines with glucose.

Given that most of the human brain, the tissue comprises fatty acid, taking omega-3 and omega-6 boosts learning and sensory execution.

In addition, ketones in a ketogenic diet help the brain to generate adenosine triphosphate (ATP), the brain particle that transmits energy for metabolism within the cells. Ketones also decrease the number of destructive cells that the body produces.

Whenever a person talks, thinks, or processes information, glutamate receptors are involved. Glutamate is a neurotransmitter that boosts stimulation in the body and is crucial in cognitive function and learning.

Glutamate should convert into GABA, but sometimes the change does not take place as successfully as it should. Therefore, ketones give an alternative source of energy that allows the brain to convert the extra glutamate into GABA efficiently.

Subsequently, the keto diet helps to increase the production of gamma-aminobutyric acid (GABA) and to reduce the number of excess neurons that fire in the brain. That helps to boost mental focus and helps to decrease the presence of stress and anxiety.

Additionally, the ketogenic diet helps to treat congenital hyperinsulinism, relieves migraine headaches, reducing the effects of Parkinson's disease, and speeds up the recovery of traumatic brain injuries.

Keto Aliments for Body Health

The ketogenic diet is an excellent means for enhancing a person's body functions by burning excess fat, balancing hormones, and reducing cravings.

Keto promotes body health by turning fat into energy and speeding up weight loss. The diet achieves this by reducing the hunger levels in a person while maintaining a healthy nutritional balance in that person's body.

Additionally, the keto diet reduces acne. When a person eats foods that are high in processed and refined carbohydrates, he or she can change gut bacteria and bring about sudden fluctuations in blood sugar, which can have an impact on skin health. Reduced carb intake can prevent the development of acne.

Fats, protein, and carbohydrates change the way the body utilizes energy, bringing about ketosis. Studies show that ketosis reduces seizures in children who experience focal seizures. Doctors advise children who have not responded to various seizure medicines to adopt a ketogenic diet.

Some of the ketogenic foods with health benefits include:

- Seafood - Fish and shellfish are healthy sources vitamins, minerals, and omega-3 fatty acids

- Low-carb vegetables - non-starchy vegetables are versatile, and they help to reduce the risk of illnesses

- Cheese is rich in calcium, protein, and healthy fatty acids with a minimal amount of carbs

- Plain yogurt and cottage cheese help to reduce appetite and promote fullness

- Avocados are rich in potassium and fiber, which improve heart function.

- Grass-fed meat and poultry are high-protein foods rich in omega-3 fatty acids, conjugated linoleic acids, and antioxidants, and are low in carbs

- Egg yolks contain lutein and zeaxanthin which help to keep the eye healthy

- Coconut oil is rich in MCTs which increase ketone production and promote loss of weight and belly fat

- Extra virgin oil is high in fats and antioxidants keeps the heart-healthy

- Nuts and seeds are high in fiber and facilitate healthier

- Berries provide nutrients that reduce the risk of disease

- Olives are rich in antioxidants that promote healthy bones

- Unsweetened tea and coffee boost the body's metabolic rate, physical and mental health

Keto Aliments for Heart Health

Keto diet helps to reduce inflammations, lower blood pressure and to increase insulin function. The diet accomplishes that by reducing the amount of fat in the body. There are two types of fats in the human body; triglycerides and cholesterol.

Triglycerides are fatty-acid molecules that reserve energy for later use. Too many triglycerides in the blood can increase the risk of getting diabetes, cardiovascular illnesses, and other life-threatening diseases.

Cholesterol is a waxy lipid produced in the liver that supports functions in the body. Such functions include building hormones, maintaining the proper functioning of cell membranes, and facilitating the absorption of vitamins. A person's body produces about 75 percent of cholesterol. The remaining 25 percent comes from animal protein.

Lipoproteins help to transport cholesterol around a person's body. The lipoproteins include the high-density lipoprotein (HDL) or the good cholesterol, and the low-density lipoprotein (LDL) or the bad cholesterol.

HDL transports cholesterol around the body, collects, and returns good cholesterol to the liver for recycling or discarding. In that way, HDL prevents cholesterol from accumulating and clogging arteries.

Unlike HDL, LDL moves slowly through the bloodstream and is vulnerable to free radicals, which are oxidizing agents. Once oxidized, LDL can quickly burrow itself into the walls of a person's artery and impede cardiovascular function. That triggers an inflammatory response in which white blood cells rush to eat up the LDL, which can cause further build-up.

Healthcare associates HDL with a lower risk of cardiovascular disease. The HDL -increasing lifestyle makes a person's heart healthier and not necessarily the drugs that raise HDL. A person can naturally raise HDL by following a ketogenic diet, which decreases LDL while increasing HDL.

Recent research shows that although higher levels of LDL can be harmful to heart health, the size, and the density of the LDL particles matter. It is essential for a person to know both the size and density of LDL particles. That is because larger LDL particles are healthier for the body.

However, while a person's diet is vital in preventing heart diseases, blood pressure, cholesterol, blood sugar, stress, smoking, and family history are factors that can contribute to the possibility of a person developing heart disease.

Therefore, if a person is at risk of developing heart disease, he or she should seek advice from a cardiologist, before he or she goes on a keto diet especially when the person has a family history of the disease.

In conclusion, the ketogenic diet helps a person to lose weight. However, it may be a short-term solution and not really a sustainable diet plan in real-life experiences. While a keto diet can help to reduce excess body fat, the goal should be to keep away the lost weight.

It is therefore advisable for a person who wishes to follow a keto diet to consult a knowledgeable health practitioner or dietician with experience in prescribing the diet plan, and in ensuring that the diet will have no adverse effects on a person.

Therefore, a person following the ketogenic diet should utilize fat wisely rather than excessively and seek nutritional ketosis rather than higher ketone levels.

Chapter 5: Types of Keto Diet Plans

A ketogenic or keto diet is one that contains a little number of carbohydrates, moderate proteins, and is high in dietary fats. The main aims of such foods are to burn body fat and reduce the levels of glucose circulating in the blood. These diets are particularly therapeutic to overweight people, people with epilepsy, and type 2 diabetics. Due to the low carbohydrates, the body learns to obtain its calories and glucose from other sources. Therefore, the liver breaks down fats into ketone bodies and fatty acids.

Dietary fats and the body's fat storage become the new sources of calories. The brain and other organs use ketone bodies as a substitute for glucose. For health reasons, the associated breakdown of fatty tissue leads to weight loss. As a result, ketogenic diets are beneficial to sufferers of obesity and other related weight loss programs. Beware of meager amounts of dietary carbohydrates and proteins since you may become underweight and stunted in growth, respectively.

Keto Starting Plan

For you to get started on a keto regimen, you need to adhere to some dietary instructions. The keto starting plan requires the creation of a food strategy based on specific guiding principles. The starting plan will act as a guideline on what to consume in your diet. It also contains details on how much you should eat, and how to manage the keto flu. The keto flu is a myriad of uncomfortable symptoms from which you may suffer when newly embarking on a ketogenic diet. Experiencing this type of flu is akin to having carbohydrate withdrawal symptoms. It is imperative to stick to specific foods for you to achieve a proper keto diet. Such keto-friendly diets will allow you to have an improved health status by enabling you to lose a significant amount of weight.

A basic rule involves keeping an eye on what you eat and knowing what to avoid. For instance, you need to cut down on starchy grains, cereals, and tubers such as potatoes. In addition, you must keep clear of sources of too much sugar, specifically honey, maple syrup, and sweet fruits. Try to seek whole foods while avoiding all forms of processed meals, as well. Your keto objectives are achievable by sticking to keto recipes when cooking meals and checking food labels for hidden carbs. Examples of the recommended foods include beef, fish, eggs, avocadoes, cheese, nuts, berries, poultry, and leafy vegetables.

The next rule concerns the quantity of food that you need to consume. After establishing the right type of keto meal, determining its precise amount is crucial in your planning.

Calories are the leading indicators of weight gain or loss, hence the need to pay attention to them. For you to attain a balance in calories, an awareness of your food quotas in addition to sticking to the correct food is essential. Gaining weight is a result of a calorie surplus, while a deficit causes an associated weight loss.

Since all human bodies treat calories as an energy source, it is almost impossible to avoid caloric diets entirely. Hence, the need to pay attention to the number of calories that you consume. Weight loss is associated with a low risk of developing diabetes and heart diseases. Thus, your objective should be to lose weight healthily by keeping your carb intake levels below thirty-five grams daily. For you to achieve this aim, you need to consume a lot of fat and an adequate amount of proteins. Both of these quotas allow you to maintain proper weight and muscle growth, respectively. In addition, you can keep track of your caloric intake by using a keto calculator or any mobile apps that can monitor calories.

Sufficient protein levels are essential for the repair and maintenance of muscle bulk. A complete lack of proteins in the diet usually leads to stunted growth and loss of muscle mass. However, too much protein is counter-productive since it can undergo gluconeogenesis, thereby impairing the much-needed ketosis. The recommended portion of your meals that are made up of protein is around twenty percent. A high-fat diet is the underlying principle of a ketogenic meal. It is the primary source of calories in any keto regimen due to the low amounts of carbohydrates in such a meal. You should strive to allocate around seventy-five percent of your diet to fats. This portion should be enough to meet the target of losing one to two pounds of weight each week.

Such excellent sources of dietary fat include eggs, avocadoes, bacon, nuts, and seeds. Beef is a highly recommended source of both protein and fat as opposed to poultry or fish, which have a high protein but zero fat level. In addition to controlling the amount of food that you consume regularly, you should develop a habit of eating when you are hungry. Besides, although exercise is not necessary, it is highly recommended in a ketogenic lifestyle. However, the light practice has to be mild and not exhaustive since you lack the high number of calories that typically come from carbs.

In the case of keto flu, you should be aware of its related symptoms and the way to remedy it. Whenever you decide to enter into a keto regimen, flu-like signs may accompany the experience. These irritable feelings are the result of your body switching from carbs as a principle source of fuel to fats. Symptoms typically develop within a few days of starting a keto diet. They include generalized fatigue, headaches, muscular cramps, and mental fogginess. Constipation and diarrhea are bowel symptoms that occur because of ketones and fat intolerance, respectively.

These last two symptoms are not necessarily part of the keto flu since poor fat tolerance is an inborn or, perhaps, a genetic condition. For you to get relief from the keto flu, you should maintain adequate hydration levels. In addition to drinking more water, you need to increase your intake of electrolytes, especially sodium, magnesium, and potassium. The high degree of ketones in the blood circulation that results from ketosis leads to constipation. However, the inclusion of leafy vegetables in your diet can remedy this condition.

Keto Basic Plan

A basic plan for a ketogenic diet involves the preparation of a sample meal that meets the targets set by a keto regimen. The objective is to have a low carb, adequate-protein, and high-fat diet. Drinking plenty of water for hydration is advisable, as well. A basic keto plan for a single week can include the following:

Monday

- Breakfast: cheese omelet, tomatoes, and eggs

- Lunch: peanut butter, almond milk, and chicken salad

- Dinner: salad, beef, and leafy vegetables

Tuesday

- Breakfast: whole milkshake or dark chocolate

- Lunch: avocadoes and fish salad in olive oil

- Dinner: consume broccoli, pork chops, and salad

Wednesday

- Breakfast: eggs, bacon, and tomatoes

- Lunch: cheese, leafy vegetables, and chicken fillet

- Dinner: asparagus, and salmon prepared in butter

Thursday

- Breakfast: mushrooms, bacon, and fried eggs

- Lunch: cheeseburger and guacamole

- Dinner: you can eat eggs and steak with salad

Friday

- Breakfast: tomatoes, cheese, and ham omelet

- Lunch: beef, vegetables, or salad with a helping of nuts and seeds

- Dinner: eggs, spinach, and whitefish

Saturday

- Breakfast: stevia, cocoa powder, and sugarless yogurt

- Lunch: fried beef and vegetables

- Dinner: you can consume an egg sandwich with cheese and bacon

Sunday

- Breakfast: avocado slices and omelet with onions

- Lunch: salsa, guacamole, celery sticks with nuts and seeds

- Dinner: cream cheese, vegetables, pork chops, and chicken salad

Keto Snack for your health

Keto snacks are useful in case you experience hunger pangs between mealtimes. The examples of keto snacks that are beneficial for your health include hard-boiled eggs, fat yogurt, strawberries, cheese, and a handful of seeds or nuts. A few pieces of fatty meat from the remaining portions of previous keto meals can function as snacks, as well.

Keto Fasting Plan

This plan involves employing intermittent fasting as a weight-loss strategy in addition to your keto diet. Skipping meals leads to a significant loss of body fat, especially during periods of weight stagnation. Other health benefits of periodic fasting include better muscle growth with strength, an enhanced level of metabolism, and increased cellular autophagy. The process of autophagy involves the cellular breakdown of unnecessary sections of itself, followed by protein recycling. Your cells, therefore, rid themselves of radical elements and toxic compounds that would otherwise accelerate the aging process or cause cancer eventually. Your mental focus and thought clarity will also show an overall improvement throughout the day. Any instances of mental fogginess and absent-mindedness disappear as well.

This strategy typically breaks down your eating habits into feeding and fasting periods. The main objective is to enable you to have a large meal in a single sitting after an extended period of hunger. A limit on your intake of calories results from intermittent fasting since the body can tolerate only a definite quantity of food at a go. Beware of snacking subconsciously during the fasting windows. After a period of adjustment to this new strategy, your body adapts to the cyclical sequence. A period of fasting enhances the process of ketosis, leading to the breakdown of your fatty tissues. Rather than look for energy from dietary fat, your body will obtain its necessary fuel from the stored body fat instead.

A famous type of intermittent fasting involves splitting the day into two sections that contain either sixteen or eight hours each. In this strategy, you can allocate the first sixteen hours to fasting, followed by the consumption of all your recommended daily calories in the remaining eight hours. Another method that you can use involves allocating the fasting and eating periods into separate days, thereby resulting in twenty-four-hour alternating windows. Intermittent keto fasting is attainable by skipping both your lunch and breakfast every day, as well.

The overarching purpose is to refrain from eating any food for a specified period consciously while being mindful of your timing strictly. However, fasting may seem challenging at first, but it is possible with proper dedication and discipline. After all, its success depends on your efforts and willingness to attain your ketogenic and weight loss objectives. Remember that fasting leads to a state of caloric deficit, thereby assisting you in achieving your aims. Although it is not essential, fasting in regular cycles is always beneficial if you want to maintain a specific weight standard. It generally leads to a refreshed feeling afterward among most people who incorporate it into their keto lifestyle.

In addition, whenever you experience the periods of fasting, your metabolic state shifts into a fat-burning mode. The liver receives instructions from the brain to begin the process of lipolysis, which generally involves breaking down fatty tissue. From this breakdown, you will have ketone bodies and fatty acids. The ketone bodies serve as fuel for the brain activities in place of the deficient glucose. As a result, the health of your nervous system gets a massive boost while preventing unwanted cases of epilepsy.

More so, fasting and the resulting ketones have an inhibitory effect on certain hormones that link to hunger. For instance, ketones inhibit the secretion and activity of the ghrelin hormone. This hormone is responsible for the sensation of hunger in humans. Its suppression eliminates the associated feelings of food cravings from your system. The inclusion of Keto-proof coffee or tea in your breakfast diet has the same hunger-suppressing effect as well as boosting your energy levels. Cortisol hormone rises in response to the increased levels of circulating ketones as well.

The high cortisol level enhances the process of muscle growth and repair. It also enables you to have a good night's sleep, especially when confronted with the keto flu. Therefore, overall, fasting led to fat breakdown and increased ketone production, which in turn, results in the suppression of hunger. All these actions and their corresponding effects give rise to a positive feedback loop that makes your intermittent fasting worthwhile eventually.

A keto calculator is a helpful tool with which you can estimate your daily macronutrient requirements. It comes in handy, especially during times of intermittent fasting. When you are still new to using the fasting strategy in your ketogenic lifestyle, you will need this calculator more than anyone will. In ketogenic fasting, you are bound to rely on hunches and guesswork on the amount of food to consume. The urge to overeat during your feeding periods may cause you to surpass the recommended daily caloric intake accidentally. A longer feeding cycle should precede your first fasting window to offset this high caloric temptation. The keto calculator uses your relevant details and any information that you feed it to compute the ideal amount of calories needed during your next meal.

Since you will have all of your data at your fingers, you must use it to keep track of your progress in the initial phases of ketogenic fasting. Certain mobile apps, such as Chronometer and MyFitnessPal, also offer services that are similar to the keto calculator. The portability factor provided by such apps comes in handy, especially in situations that render you to somewhat unfamiliar surroundings. Another essential point to keep in mind is not to engage in any snacking. Snacks are meals too, albeit tiny amounts, and hence they will defeat the purpose of fasting.

A sample meal during the feeding phase of a regular keto fasting cycle could look like this:

- **Breakfast:** Keto-proof green tea or coffee. Remember that this drink contains a mixture of dietary fats and oils within it. This fatty mixture is justified as long as you can avoid any form of carbs.

- **Lunch:** Black coffee, water, and sugarless tea. This lunch is ideally a fasting period that allows you to consume lots of water and other fluids. The resulting improvement in hydration serves to mitigate any adverse effects from the keto flu.

- **Dinner:** Consume your meals as per the ketogenic diet and follow the dinner examples shown earlier within the basic plans.

Keto Vegetarian Plan

The combination of a vegetarian diet with a ketogenic one is often doubly beneficial to your overall health status. Both heart diseases and problems related to increased weight are preventable using this vegetarian keto diet. You end up keeping conditions such as obesity and diabetes at bay effectively. Unlike the vegan keto diet, a vegetarian one allows you to consume animal products without the need for the real animal or its flesh. Your diet should have the usual limitation to its carbohydrate contents to below thirty-five grams daily. The incorporation of eggs and dairy is standard in such foods.

The widespread reasons for embarking on a vegetarian diet share a common thread. The common ground relates to environmental preservation, curbing climate change, sustainability, and eliminating cases of animal torture. Losing weight and attaining better health are often novelty reasons for including a ketogenic component to the diet. Restricting your animal products to free-range livestock is an extra step that you can take to ensure adherence to your ethos. Controlled animals are likely to face exposure to fattening hormonal injections and chemical treatments that are detrimental to your health in the end.

Remember that your keto diet should contain high-fat sources to make up for the low quantities of carbs while sticking to your vegetarian principles. Your sources of dietary fat are plenty in spite of a lack of fatty beef, pork chops, bacon, or steak. Eggs, high-fat dairy products, and plant-based fats can make up the difference. The inclusion of micronutrient and multivitamin supplements in your diet is advisable, too, since you may not get all the recommended nutrients from plant sources alone.

Consuming plenty of low-carb vegetables such as asparagus, celery, zucchini, and leafy spinach is also preferable. In case you run into challenges when trying to estimate the number of calories you need to include in the diet, use a keto calculator. It works in the same manner across all forms of keto diets to keep your intake of calories within the recommended limits.

Keto Vegan Plan

A vegan diet is devoid of any animals or their products as the primary source of protein. Due to the highly restrictive nature of a vegan ketogenic diet, you will need tremendous willpower to pull it off successfully. In this case, you may have to combine a typical ketogenic diet with high-carb vegan sources to meet your daily caloric quota. Such a vegan keto diet contains many low-carb vegetables limited to thirty-five grams daily, as well as many plant-based fats and proteins. Multivitamin supplements are beneficial to account for the vitamin deficiency that is common in vegan bodies.

For you to know how much fats and proteins, you will require from the plant sources, you need to use the keto calculator as well. Keep in mind that your diet will be entirely void of fish, poultry, beef, eggs, dairy, and any other animal products. However, you can use meat substitutes such as tofu and soy products in some instances. Mushrooms, leafy vegetables, nuts, and seeds also provide a low-carb source of calories. Avocadoes and berries contained in the regular keto diet are safe within a vegan setting, as well. Dairy products in a particular vegan diet are replaceable with coconut milk and cream. In addition, coconut oil and butter are useful in cooking and frying specific foods within this category. Beware of the lower melting point of the coconut oil over its butter equivalent.

You can choose from a variety of vegan cheese in the market nowadays. Based on your preference, vegan cheese replaces the need for dairy sources efficiently. You can easily substitute ground flax seeds for poultry eggs to obtain a credible vegan keto diet. Other available substitutes for eggs include silken tofu, baking soda, and vinegar. Examples of plant-based sources of fat include avocadoes, coconut oils, olive oils, seeds, coconut butter, and most nuts. This diet is often pointless for people who are unfortunate to suffer from neural ailments such as epilepsy, Alzheimer's, and Parkinson's diseases. The epileptic nature of these brain conditions is manageable using a ketogenic diet via the production of therapeutic ketones.

Chapter 6: The Information You Must Know About Keto Cycling

Keto diet is a low-carb, moderate protein, and high-fat diet, which has several variations. Keto cycling is one of the less restrictive keto diet variations that allow one to have a day of eating carbs. People who follow a keto diet eat under 50 grams of carbs per day. This enables their bodies to switch from using carbs as a primary source of fuel to using fat, a process known as ketosis.

What Is a Cyclical Keto Diet?

For a cyclical keto diet, an individual would need to follow a strict low-carb, high-fat diet for five to six days a week, and then have a high carb once or twice in a week, which is essentially a cheat day. When you follow a cyclical keto diet, it removes the body out of ketosis for one or two days and goes back into ketosis thereafter for the rest of the week until your next cheat day. The high-carb eating day also known as the refeeding day replenishes the body's glucose reserves. This helps improve muscle growth as well as exercise performance.

The Way to Equilibrate Cycles of Keto Diet

It is possible to cycle on and off a keto diet. Some people feel great eating a low-carb diet and can maintain it for a long period however; some give it a shot but find it hard to stick by it. Instead of quitting altogether, there are ways you can adjust to an on and off-cycle and still enjoy the health benefits. You can experiment and tweak your keto diet until you find what works best for you. You can equilibrate cycles of the keto diet in the following three ways:

1. The moderate carb approach

This approach allows you to increase your daily carb approach from the normal 50 grams to about 150 grams per day and reduce your high fat intake. The extra carbs should be from healthy carb options like brown rice, baked yams, sweet potatoes, or fruits. The fats should also be from healthy sources like nuts, avocado, olive oil or seeds. This approach is perfect for people who prefer a slightly higher carb intake. The increase in carbs promotes a person's sleep pattern.

2. The weekly keto cycling approach

Another approach you can use to avoid going off keto entirely is to cycle your carb intake throughout the week. Follow a strict 50 grams low carb diet for five to six days then increase your carb intake up to 155 grams for one or two days and then go back to the low-carb keto diet. This approach works well for people who need help to jump-start their metabolism.

3. The seasonal keto approach

This approach works well for people who cannot follow a keto diet full time or those who need to adjust to in-season foods. Some people may want to follow a keto diet maybe once or twice a year to reap its benefits for a short period, and then go back to normal eating. Athletes cannot follow a keto diet full time but can follow it off-season.

Keto Cycle Program

To start on a cyclical keto diet,

1. **It is best to follow a keto diet for at least a month before starting keto cycling.**

Follow the standard keto diet for four to six weeks. That way your body gets time to adjust to the keto diet and you can drift on and off ketosis as you like. When your body is used to ketosis, it usually reverts to ketosis faster after having a high-carb day.

2. **Follow the standard keto diet (SKD) for five to six days a week**

During that period consumes less than 50 grams of carbs a day and increase the amount of healthy fats intake. Such fats include avocado, eggs, coconut oil, olive oil, nuts, and seeds. Choose healthy sources of protein like salmon, fish, poultry, or lean beef. Avoid processed meat like sausages and bacon. Ensure you follow a meal plan of 75% fat, 20% protein, and only 5% carbs. Avoid sugary foods, grains, fruits, root vegetables, and tubers.

3. Have a high carb cheat day

Choose a day or two when you can indulge in high carbs to get the body out of ketosis and replenish glucose levels. Don't have a whole pizza or burger and fries, stick to healthy carbs like brown rice, beans, quinoa, lentils, oats, or sweet potatoes. Pair the meal with moderate protein.

4. Go Back to Ketosis

After the refeeding days, go back to your standard keto diet. To achieve ketosis faster, you can either practice:

- **Intermittent Fasting** - This is time-restricted feeding where you have meals within a short period of six hours and fast for the remaining 18 hours of the day. Intermittent fasting helps the body transition smoothly in and out of ketosis.

- **High-Intensity Workouts** - On the days following refeeding, go for high-intensity workouts, which help burn the excess carbs consumed.

Benefits of Keto Cycling

1. Weight loss

When you reduce carbs and increase fat intake, the body enters a metabolic state called ketosis. Ideally, the body uses carbs as the main source of energy but during ketosis, because very little carbs are consumed, the body is forced to use fat as a source of energy. After a few days of following the diet, the body starts burning fat for fuel causing weight loss.

2. Muscle building

Some studies have revealed that going on Keto cycling can help those who want to lose weight and gain muscle. Healthy carbs are good for building muscles. The keto cycle usually prevents the production of muscle-building hormones like insulin. However, with the on and off ketosis days, you regulate insulin production, which promotes muscle gain.

3. Reduces full-on Keto side effects

When you follow any keto diet, you are likely to experience serious side effects. This may include headaches, nausea, weakness, fatigue and sometimes lack of sleep. When you break the full-on Keto diet with a day or two of indulging in a high carb, it decreases these symptoms because you are not in ketosis for so many days at once.

4. Makes the diet more sustainable

Keto diets cut down on all types of carbs, which normally account for at least 50% of what the majority of people eat. Because it is so restrictive, it is really hard to follow through the long term. When you use the cyclical keto diet, you have days you can eat carbs, therefore making the diet more sustainable.

5. Boost performance

Studies have revealed that athletes who followed a cyclical keto diet performed better compared to those following a standard keto diet.

6. Reduces the negative effects

When on a full keto diet, people don't indulge in carbs and according to some studies, this carb restriction over a long period has a negative impact on hormones, cholesterol levels, and mood swings. But with regular replenishment using keto cycling, these problems are avoided.

7. Better Insulin Sensitivity

When you go for the five days on a low carb diet, your body becomes more sensitive to insulin. However, prolonged periods of a low carb diet can make the body insensitive to insulin and cause weight gain. Keto cycling ensures that you don't stay on a low carb diet for too long to cause such effects.

The Difference Between Keto Cycling and Carb Cycling

While both involve eating fewer carbs, keto cycling follows a high fat, moderate protein and lower carb diet and carb cycling follows a high-protein, moderate fat and just cuts down on carbs for a few days. With carb cycling, the body does not have to switch to burning fat for fuel.

Keto cycling allows one to have high carbs once or twice a week to replenish glucose levels while in carb cycling you alternate your carb intake on a daily, weekly, or monthly basis. The goal is to train the body not to rely solely on carbs for energy but also to use fat as an alternative source of fuel. Most people who follow carb cycling are athletes because it helps enhance their performance and maximize energy stores for competition.

In carb cycling, you can program your carb intake based on your routine. You can have high carbs on days you do high-intensity workouts and muscle building days and eat low carbs on your rest days. While in keto cycling, the high carb days are fixed. If you have carbs on Saturdays, you should have them on all other consecutive Saturdays. Carb cycling typically prevents the negative impacts of a low carb diet experienced on a keto cycling.

Is Keto Cycling Good for You? (Advantages and Disadvantages)

The jury is still out on whether keto cycling is good or bad. It all boils down to an individual's preferred dietary choices. If you feel keto cycling is helping you stay on track, then go for it and if you also feel like keto cycling is challenging and is making you overindulge on those refeeding days, then do not do it.

Women who are pregnant or nursing should not follow Keto cycling or any keto diet. Patients with type 2 diabetes need to consult their doctors beforehand but those with type 1 diabetes should not follow a keto diet. Keto cycling is a good way to help you stick to the keto diet in the end however; it is also too unbalanced and restrictive. It restricts a person from eating certain food items regularly, which are important.

Advantages

1. Losing weight

Many people follow keto cycling to lose weight. Research has shown that people lose weight faster when they go on keto diets. Without glucose from carbs, your body burns stored fat as fuel.

2. Curbs inflammations

You use fat as fuel as opposed to carbs it causes far less inflammation. The fat breaks down into ketones, which also reduces the inflammatory response.

3. Keeps you fuller for longer

A Keto cycling diet keeps you full for longer because ketones regulate the hormones responsible for hunger. When you are hungry, your body will just burn stored fat to keep you going.

4. Good for the brain

On the five or six days that you are on ketosis, the brain benefits a lot. It uses ketones for energy to make more mitochondria and with more mitochondria; your cells generate more energy.

Disadvantages

1. Difficult to Sustain

Even though Keto cycling allows for carbs intake once or twice a week, it still restricts too many important food groups and even though people do lose weight, the majority gains it back when they resume their carb intake.

2. Weight fluctuations

People experience weight fluctuations when they transition from a full-on keto diet to a cyclical keto diet. This is because their bodies retain excess water when high-carb foods are consumed. So, during refeeding, they will gain weight and when they are back to ketosis, the weight goes back down.

3. Binge Eating

People who follow the keto cycling will maintain a low-carb diet for the five or six days but on the refeeding day, they indulge in as many carbohydrates as they want which counteracts the weight loss benefits of any keto diet. That restriction on carbs can lead to bingeing.

4. Your body might store more fat

When you eat a high-fat diet and then switch to high carbs, you can be in danger of storing much of the consumed fat. The body might use the carbs as energy, stop converting fat to energy, and therefore store the fat.

5. Keto can lead to high cholesterol

Keto follows a high-fat diet. If a person does not avoid bad fats like saturated fats or Trans fats, they can lead to high cholesterol levels, heart diseases, and stroke. Fat consumed during keto should have good cholesterol levels. People on a keto diet should stick to plant-based unsaturated fats like avocados, nuts, and seeds.

Conclusion

Thank you for making it through to the end of *Keto Diet for Beginners: An Ultimate Keto Diet Guide for Beginners Code to Use Keto Aliments, Alkaline Plant and Vegetable to Eliminate Obesity and Weight Loss Fast Improve Your Health Eating Healthy Food*. Let us hope it was informative and able to provide you with all of the tools you need to achieve your goals whatever they may be.

Now you know that the word keto comes from the fact that this diet plan drives the body to produce ketones, which are tiny energy/fuel molecules. The body turns to this fuel source when the level of blood sugar is low. The keto diet plan has its origins date back to the 1920s as a treatment plan for childhood epilepsy. According to some studies, people who follow this diet experience up to 40% fewer epileptic seizures.

Ketosis is the state where ketone bodies build up in the bloodstream. When the body reaches ketosis, metabolism switches to fat-burning to convert accumulated fat molecules into ketone bodies, which help power the brain and muscles. Being in a state of ketosis, therefore, sounds like an awesome way to get rid of excess fat.

A research done in 2007 showed that a low carb diet was effective in controlling blood pressure. This is because keto diet helps in reducing body mass, LDL cholesterol, and triglycerides. In September 2016, the Journal of Obesity and Eating Disorders published research suggesting that the keto diet could be helpful to people with type 2 diabetes and lead to improvements in the levels of HbA1c.

According to one study published in the journal Endocrine in December 2016, obese people on a low-calorie keto diet lose ore inflammatory belly fat as compared to those on a normal low-calorie diet. Experts such as Robert Krikorian, Ph.D., a professor of clinical psychiatry, are conducting studies looking at whether inducing dietary ketosis can preserve cognitive functioning.

Some studies, such as one published in the journal Oncology in November 2018; suggest that doctors should use the ketogenic diet in conjunction with radiation and chemotherapy to treat certain forms of cancer. According to some experts in the field of neuroscience, some of the effects induced by the keto diet may include GABA neurotransmission and enhanced purinergic, sensitive potassium channel modulation, and boosted brain-derived neurotrophic factor expression because of glycolytic limitation.

There are different types of fats: bad ones and good ones. Monounsaturated fats and polyunsaturated are healthy fats. These fats come from vegetables, nuts, fish, and seeds. The bad fats include the industrial made Trans fats that come in solid kinds of margarine and vegetable shortening while the saturated fats are neither good nor bad and they mostly come from animal products like meat and whole milk.

The Keto diet involves taking 75% high-fat food, 20% protein, and only 5% carbs. After a few days of observing this percentage of foods in your diet, your body will get into a state called ketosis whereby the body burns stored fat in the body.

When a person eliminates carbs from his or her diet, ketones can give up to 70 percent of the brain's energy. However, that means that the body is still getting 20 to 25 percent of its energy from glucose.

The keto starting plan requires the creation of a food strategy based on specific guiding principles. The starting plan will act as a guideline on what to consume in your diet. It also contains details on how much you should eat, and how to manage the keto flu.

The next step is to try out the Keto diet for you to start enjoying the benefits of great health and manageable weight.

Finally, if you found this book useful in any way, a review on Amazon is always appreciated!

www.ingramcontent.com/pod-product-compliance
Lightning Source LLC
Chambersburg PA
CBHW031236250726
48655CB00005B/1977